CNA Prac

CNA Nursing Assistant - Practice Classes 1

32 Practice Classes plus Quizzes

CNA Registry at **www.CNAClasses.US**

VoicesNet Media Publishing

A Division of VoicesNet Media, LLC

Copyright 2014

Published in Powell, Ohio by VoicesNet Media, LLC.

Library of Congress Cataloging-in-Publication Data

VoicesNet Media Publishing

CNA Nursing Assistant Practice Classes 1

From the CNA Registry at CNAClasses.US

ISBN 10: 0976681005 ISBN 13: 978-0976681007

Training   Healthcare   Classes

Printed in the United States of America

Table of Contents

Introduction

We are the CNA Registry at CNAClasses.US. We have been around since 2009 and are operated by VoicesNet Media, LLC.

Our Founder and CEO is Jeff Humphrey. He has set up an electronic network of training and communication that is helping caregivers become better at taking care of their clients/patients.

Caregivers trained by the material in this book and at the CNAClasses.US website are better able to get their industry and job certifications.

This book is comprised of 32 caregiver mini-courses followed by small multiple choice quizzes for each course. It will help someone prepare for caregiver training and caregiver jobs. It's another tool to improve your education.

The CNA Registry at CNAClasses.US provides free and premium online caregiver classes to the general public and to organizations. We also provide CNA certification information for all fifty states. We serve an average of 20,000 online courses per month.

Students from all across the United States have benefited from the information provided. As of this book publication, we currently have over 32,000 members in our CNA caregiver registry.

Caregiver organizations are now using our training material and software to train their staffs.

As of this book publication, there are over 55 free online CNA/Caregiver practice classes and 172 total classes at CNAClasses.US, complete with quizzes.

Book Dedication

I would like to personally thank the people involved in creating this book.

First of all, this book is dedicated to all of the wonderful caregivers who are giving their all to take care of those who are not able to completely take care of themselves. You inspire us to create training books like this.

Caregivers exhibit love and compassion and are the framework of care in the healthcare system. They are called CNAs, HHAs, PCAs, Caregivers and many other names. They are often called Angels.

Many caregivers have come to www.CNAClasses.US over the last few years to train and improve their lives. We are thankful and humbled to be a part of their journey and to have them become a part of ours.

The content in this book was written by multiple healthcare educators over a number of years. We would like to thank all of the nurses and nursing aides who previously contributed to this material.

A great "thank you" goes out to Jackie Humphrey, who worked as the Curriculum Coordinator during the many editing rounds that this book and its creators endured. Jackie was the hub who worked with company management, the editors, and the nurses, to produce this wonderful book.

To our nurse writers, who always perform at a very high professional level, we thank you so much. Lead nurse writer Vivian Alsup, and our other nurse writers, Suzanne Ball, and Pat Bratianu, have created some tremendous material for this book and the CNAClasses.US website.

Also, Mercy Pilkington, owner of Author Options, was critical to the project's success and should be thanked for her deep knowledge of grammar and style and also for reviewing and editing the manuscript.

Jeff Humphrey

COURSE # 1 - ADL - Bathing, Dressing, & Grooming

You are assigned to dress a rehab patient who doesn't like to assist you in dressing. To try to get her cooperation, you should:

Explain to the patient that showing she can help will play a part in being able to go home.

Rationale: Rehab patients aren't discharged home until the doctor feels the patients can safely perform all of the activities of daily living by themselves or with very minimal help. Getting dressed is a basic activity that the patients must be able to do independently before being discharged.

When bathing a patient, you should not:

Leave the patient to answer a call light

Rationale: Patients who need help bathing often feel embarrassed or ashamed, and privacy should be respected. Communicate with the patient and tell him what you will be washing next. Cover the patient with a bath blanket and only expose the body part being washed. Never leave the patient alone in the middle of bathing. Instead, have someone else answer your call lights while you are bathing your patient.

Mouth care should be performed on a patient:

Several times a day

Rationale: Mouth care should be provided for patients every morning, afternoon, and evening. This is often overlooked, but is one of the most important parts of patient care. Mouth care includes brushing the teeth, wiping the mouth, using mouthwash, and possibly even flossing. Oral swabs should be used for patients who have no teeth, who take nothing by mouth, or who are not conscious.

You are dressing a patient with right arm weakness. The side that you start dressing first is:

The right side

Rationale: Because the patient's right arm is weak and she won't be able to assist as much with that side, start with that side first because it will be easier to maneuver. She will be able to assist you in putting her left arm through a sleeve hole much more easily. This will be the most comfortable for the patient, too.

Patients should be bathed:

Every day

Rationale: Patients should be bathed every day. This includes either a shower or bed bath. Clean skin prevents infection and skin breakdown, and promotes confidence in patients. Patients usually have an assigned shower schedule which may only allow for two to three showers a week, so bed baths will keep patients clean between showers.

The patient's hair should be brushed:

After getting her ready for the day

Rationale: A patient's hair should be brushed every morning after she is dressed for the day or after a shower. Keeping a patient well-groomed can help her feel confident and want to socialize with other patients. If it is not a shower day, dampen the hair and gently comb it to prevent pulling.

Peri-care should be provided:

During bathing and after each episode of incontinence

Rationale: Peri-care prevents patients from getting urinary tract infections, yeast infections, and skin breakdown. It should be performed each time a patient is bathed and after each episode of bowel and/or bladder incontinence. Nursing assistants can use a washing cloth with gentle soap and warm water, or with a special wipe made specifically for peri-care.

The following should be done after a patient is bathed:

Put lotion on the patient to prevent any dryness or skin breakdown

Rationale: Unless there is a restriction, lotion should always be put on a patient after bathing to prevent skin breakdown. Never send the patient to an activity in a robe or gown unless it is his wish to go that way, and never leave him alone in the bathroom unless he is an independent patient.

The best way to get a patient to participate in getting dressed is:

Let him make decisions about what to wear

Rationale: Patients will cooperate best and be more helpful in getting dressed if they can make decisions about what to wear and how to put on the clothes. Threatening them or doing the work for them does not foster independence.

The following is NOT appropriate when bathing a patient:

Using the same washcloth throughout the bath

Rationale: Several washcloths should be used during bathing to prevent the spreading of bacteria to openings in the body, such as the mouth or genital area. Using a bath blanket to provide privacy is a must, covering all areas of the body that aren't currently being washed. When bathing, start with the face first and work your way down, leaving the peri-area for last.

----- COURSE TEST -----

1. You are assigned to dress a rehab patient who doesn't like to assist with dressing. To try and gain the patient's cooperation, you should:

A. Explain to him that showing he can help will help him be able to go home

B. Just dress him and move on to the next patient

C. Tell him he has to help dress himself or else he doesn't get to participate in any activities today

D. Sit and wait until he decides he wants to help you

XXXXXAXXXXX

2. When bathing a patient, you should NOT do which of the following?

A. Provide privacy

B. Inform the patient of what you will be doing

C. Leave the patient to answer a call light

D. Test the water (or ask the patient to, if possible) before beginning

XXXXXCXXXXX

3. Mouth care should be performed on a patient:

A. Every morning

B. Several times a day

C. Before bed

D. When you have free time

XXXXXBXXXXX

4. You are dressing a patient with right arm weakness. Which side do you start dressing first?

A. The left side

B. It doesn't matter

C. The right side

D. Ask the patient and let her decide

XXXXXCXXXXX

5. How often should a patient be bathed?

A. Twice a week

B. Every day

C. Once weekly

D. Every other day

XXXXXBXXXXX

6. A patient's hair should be brushed:

A. After getting her ready for the day

B. Before lunch

C. Before dinner

D. Before bed

XXXXXAXXXXX

7. Peri-care should be provided how often?

A. Three times a day

B. Every morning

C. During bathing and after each episode of incontinence

D. After each episode of incontinence and at bedtime

XXXXXCXXXXX

8. Which of the following should be done after a patient is bathed?

A. Take the patient into the dirty utility room with you while you dispose of her towels

B. Send the patient to the activity room in her robe while you change her sheets

C. Leave the patient in the bathroom while you get her clothes

D. Put lotion on the patient to prevent any dryness or skin breakdown

XXXXXDXXXXX

9. What is the best way to get a patient to participate in getting dressed?

A. Let him make decisions about what to wear

B. Do most of the work for him

C. Tell him he has to help or he will be stuck there forever

D. Wait until he does it for himself

XXXXXAXXXXX

10. Which of the following is NOT appropriate when bathing a patient?

A. Using a bath blanket to cover areas not being washed

B. Using the same washcloth throughout the bath

C. Having the patient check the water to make sure it is warm enough

D. Washing the face first

XXXXXBXXXXX

COURSE # 2 - ADL - Bowel & Bladder

You should check your patients for incontinence:

Every two hours

Rationale: Because you should be rounding on your patients and checking on them every two hours, this is the best time to check to see if they have been incontinent of bowel or bladder. Urine is acidic, and the longer it remains touching the skin, the greater the chance a patient has of skin breakdown. If needed, patients should be changed more often, but some may only need to be changed a few times a day.

The purpose of bladder training is:

A way for patients to manage urinary incontinence

Rationale: Bladder training is a way for patients to learn to manage urinary incontinence. This lengthens the amount of time between bathroom trips, expands the bladder so it can hold more urine, and improves the patients' urge to urinate. The training must be strictly followed according to the program the physician sets up or else it will not work.

Your patient tells you that she hasn't had a bowel movement in three days and feels like she needs to go but she can't. You tell the nurse this patient:

Has constipation

Rationale: Constipation is irregular bowel movements or having difficulty passing stool. This can be painful and frustrating for patients. Let the nurse know you think the patient may be constipated so the nurse can assess the patient and treat her accordingly. Constipation can be dangerous for some patients, especially those who just had surgery, as straining can cause the incision to open up.

You are providing peri-care to a female patient who just had a bowel movement in her adult brief. When you wipe, you should:

Wipe front to back

Rationale: When providing peri-care for a female, always wipe the patient front to back. Stool contains E. coli, and if a patient is wiped incorrectly, E. coli can be wiped into the female's urethra. E. coli is the most common organism causing urinary tract infections, which can develop into much worse conditions and be very expensive to treat.

It is NOT appropriate when collecting a urine specimen:

To have the nurse put the label on the urine collection bottle

Rationale: When collecting urine, wipe the patient from front to back first to remove dead skin. Then have the patient start urinating in the toilet, and then begin urinating in the cup, if possible. When finished, label the urine with the patient's name and date of birth, or according to your facility's policy. Only the person collecting the specimen should label it. Refrigerate the urine immediately unless you have specific instructions not to do so.

The following is an abnormal finding when a patient urinates:

Amber urine

Rationale: Amber urine occurs when a patient is dehydrated or the kidneys are not working properly. This dark-colored urine should alert the nursing assistant that something is wrong with the patient and the nurse should be notified immediately of this finding. This may be a normal finding for a patient with known kidney disease, but if it is new, the longer it goes on means the longer it will take for the patient's kidney function to return to normal, if at all.

You notice that your patient's stools are black and tarry. You should notify the nurse of this immediately because:

The patient could be bleeding internally

Rationale: Black, tarry stools are a major sign that a patient is bleeding somewhere in the intestines and, if left untreated, will lead to death. Medications like iron can cause stools to look like this also, but it is expected then and is considered a normal medication reaction in that case. Do not assume that the patient is on iron. Inform the nurse in order to let her decide the next course of action.

You notice that a patient who was previously continent is now having frequent episodes of incontinence. You should:

Notify the nurse

Rationale: Although increased incontinence can be normal, other factors may cause this. Diseases of the bladder or intestines, abuse, social problems, and more can cause a previously continent patient to suddenly be unable to control his bladder. The nurse will investigate further and let you know if an adult brief is necessary or not.

A patient tells you that it burns every time he urinates and sometimes his urine is reddish in color. You should tell the nurse immediately because you know this is a sign of:

Urinary tract infection

Rationale: Burning sensation, frequent urination, dark urine, or blood in the urine are all signs of a urinary tract infection. Patients should be treated for this quickly to prevent it from spreading to the bladder, or worse. If left untreated, this infection can spread into the blood and cause sepsis, or can cause the kidneys to fail. Notify the nurse immediately if any of these signs are present in your patients.

You have a patient who is constipated. You should provide him with fluids to drink:

More often than before

Rationale: Extra fluids can help the patient move his bowels easier because it may moisten the stool. When constipated, a patient's stool is usually dry and hard, making it painful to pass through the rectum. Extra fluids can assist with this. You should report any complaints or signs of constipation to the nurse so she can also assist the patient with this problem by medicating him with a stool softener.

----- COURSE TEST -----

1. How often should you check your patients for incontinence?

A. Every shift

B. Every two hours

C. Every six hours

D. Every thirty minutes

XXXXXBXXXXX

2. The purpose of bladder training is:

A. A way for patients to manage urinary incontinence

B. Teaching your patients to urinate at certain hours so nursing assistants won't have to change all patients at the same time

C. To wean the bladder off of a suprapubic catheter

D. A program that teaches patients how to prevent incontinence in the future

XXXXXAXXXXX

3. Your patient tells you that she hasn't had a bowel movement in three days and feels like she needs to go but she can't. You tell the nurse this patient:

A. Has diarrhea

B. Has a bowel obstruction

C. Has constipation

D. Needs surgery

XXXXXCXXXXX

4. You are providing peri-care to a female patient who just had a bowel movement in her adult brief. When you wipe, you should:

A. Wipe front to back

B. Wipe back to front

C. Wipe side to side

D. Wipe in whatever manner gets the patient the cleanest

XXXXXAXXXXX

5. Which of the following is NOT appropriate when collecting a urine specimen?

A. Wiping the patient before urination begins to remove dead skin

B. Allowing the patient to urinate a little in the toilet first, and then into the cup

C. Refrigerating the urine

D. Having the nurse label the urine collected

XXXXXDXXXXX

6. The following is an abnormal finding when a patient urinates:

A. Yellow urine

B. Clear urine

C. Amber urine

D. Urine warm in temperature

XXXXXCXXXXX

7. You notice that your patient's stools are black and tarry. You should notify the nurse of this immediately because:

A. It is a sign of having a reaction to medication

B. He could be bleeding internally

C. He will soon become constipated

D. He has an intestinal parasite

XXXXXBXXXXX

8. You notice a patient who was previously continent is having frequent episodes of incontinence. You should:

A. Notify the nurse

B. Start placing adult briefs on the patient

C. Tell the patient she must go to the bathroom every hour to prevent this

D. Ignore this because the patient is getting older and it is probably normal

XXXXXAXXXXX

9. A patient tells you that it burns every time he urinates, and sometimes his urine is reddish in color. You should tell the nurse immediately because you know this is a sign of:

A. Bladder cancer

B. Prostate problems

C. Urinary tract infection

D. Kidney disease

XXXXXCXXXXX

10. You have a patient who is constipated. You should provide her with fluids to drink:

A. Less often than before

B. As often as before

C. Only after the constipation has subsided

D. More often than before

XXXXXDXXXXX

COURSE # 3 - ADL - Eating, Nutrition, & Hydration

You are assigned to feed a patient who gets her food pureed. The meal tray arrives and it has not been pureed. You should:

Send it back and ask the kitchen to puree it

Rationale: Patients are on pureed diets to prevent them from choking. Because patients are weak and/or unable to chew, pureed diets will essentially do the chewing for them to prevent large pieces of food from getting stuck in the esophagus and choking the patient.

You are setting up a meal tray for a patient who had a stroke and has left-sided weakness. You should set the eating utensils:

On the right side

Rationale: Utensils should be used by the strong hand, and when a nursing assistant sets up the meal, she should place them on the strong side. Physical therapy may eventually want the patient to use the affected side, but unless otherwise instructed, set up the utensils on the unaffected side.

The nurse informs you that your patient is on aspiration precautions. You know this effects how the patient eats because:

He is at risk for choking

Rationale: Patients on aspiration precautions are at risk for choking on their food and drink and inhaling them into the lungs, which leads to pneumonia and even death. The patients should be fed slowly while they are sitting up, and be on thickened liquids. If the nursing assistant has any concerns or questions, she should ask the nurse for advice.

You are taking care of a patient who isn't able to sit up to take a drink. You should check on him and offer him a drink:

Every one to two hours

Rationale: Because you should be checking on your patients every one to two hours, ask this patient during rounds if he would like a drink of water during this time. Make sure the water is cold and fresh.

You are collecting meal trays and notice that your patient didn't eat much dinner. You should:

Ask the patient if she would like a different meal

Rationale: Good nutrition is an important part of a patient's healing process. Proteins play a vital role in the healing process, and without eating, many of these proteins are not available for the body to use. The patient may simply not like the food provided and would like a different meal. Never take the meal away if it wasn't eaten and simply disregard the fact that the patient didn't eat.

You should pass out fresh water and ice to your patients:

Every eight hours

Rationale: Fresh water and ice should be passed out every eight hours or sooner if the patient's pitcher is empty and he requests more. Ideally, fresh water and ice should be passed every four to six hours, but it must be passed every eight hours to prevent the growth of bacteria and particles in the water.

Your patient ate all of the main course and one side dish. He still has one side dish leftover and doesn't want it. You record that the patient ate this much:

75%

Rationale: Facilities generally count 0, 25, 50, 75, and 100%. In this case, the main course would count for 50% and each side dish 25%. Since only one side dish was consumed, 75% of the meal was eaten. Check your facility's policies for specifics on intake documentation.

You see that your patient is on a NAS diet. You know that this means:

There should be no added salt

Rationale: NAS, or no added sodium, is for patients with cardiac problems, kidney disease, and/or high blood pressure. Sodium attracts fluids and can cause fluid overload, high blood pressure, and more. The amount of sodium should be restricted to two grams per day.

Your patient is diagnosed with dehydration. You should make the following change in the amount of fluid consumed daily:

Offer your patient a drink more frequently than normal

Rationale: Dehydration is caused by a number of things, but as part of treatment, a patient should consume a lot of fluids. Because she will need to drink more than patients who aren't dehydrated, she should be offered water more often. Do not force the patient to drink or threaten that she won't get better. If the patient continually refuses the water, tell the nurse so she can be educated on it being part of her treatment.

You are assigned to help a patient eat dinner and notice that her beverages must be thickened. This is because:

Thin liquids can cause the patient to choke

Rationale: Patients who are at risk for choking or aspirating their drinks are put on thickened liquids to prevent that from happening. Thickener comes in powder and liquid form and can be mixed with any beverage.

Your diabetic patient asks for an evening snack. Because he is a diabetic, you know the best snack for him is:

Almonds

Rationale: Many kinds of nuts are a great snack for diabetics. They are filling and low in sugar. Cookies, pudding, ice cream, and pie are full of sugar and should be avoided as a snack for a diabetic. If you are unsure of a good snack idea, ask your nurse for further advice.

You are assigned to take care of a patient with cancer who is being treated with chemotherapy. You know that his eating habits and appetite will:

Decrease

Rationale: Chemotherapy patients lose their appetite because the treatment makes them nauseous and tired. They generally eat little at meals, or not at all. Do not force them to eat if they are ill. If they are nauseous, let the nurse know and she may be able to give them medicine to help with nausea so they are able to eat.

The following is NOT appropriate when feeding a patient:

Feeding him in ten minutes so you have a chance to feed all of your patients

Rationale: When feeding a patient, you should never rush because this can cause the patient to choke or just give up on trying to eat. Meal time should be a pleasant experience. Feeding patients can take a while, especially if they are weak or tired and chew slowly. Ask for assistance in feeding your other patients if you are running behind.

You are getting a new patient on the unit who has a PEG tube. You know that you won't need to feed this patient because:

He will be fed by a nurse through the tube

Rationale: Patients with PEG tubes are fed a special mixture of liquid nutrients through their tubes. Only a nurse can set up the tube feedings, and a machine regulates how much they get and how often. These are usually given to patients who aren't able to eat through their mouths and can be either temporary or permanent. It is important to remember to still give oral care to these patients.

The nurse tells you that one of the patients on your assignment is NPO. This means:

She isn't allowed to have anything to eat or drink

Rationale: Patients who are NPO should consume nothing by mouth until the physician says they may. Patients are generally NPO before surgery, if they are intubated, or if they have a feeding tube. Their mouths may be swabbed with a moist swab, and ice chips may be allowed. NPO patients are not allowed to consume food or drink beverages.

----- COURSE TEST -----

1. You are assigned to feed a patient who gets her food pureed. Her meal tray arrives and it has not been pureed. You should:

A. Feed the food to the patient slowly

B. Mash the food up yourself

C. Send it back and ask the kitchen to puree it

D. See if the patient can eat the food whole. If not, send it back

XXXXXCXXXXX

2. You are setting up a meal tray for a patient who had a stroke and has left-sided weakness. You should set the eating utensils:

A. On the right side

B. On the left side

C. In front of the plate

D. Behind the plate

XXXXXAXXXXX

3. The nurse informs you that your patient is on aspiration precautions. You know this effects how the patient eats because:

A. He is only allowed to have a minimum amount of fluids with his meal

B. He is at risk for choking

C. He must eat all of his food in order to meet the daily nutrition requirement

D. He is at risk for vomiting after eating

XXXXXBXXXXX

4. You are taking care of a patient who isn't able to sit up to take a drink. How often should you check to see if she would like a drink?

A. Once per shift

B. Every three to four hours

C. Every thirty minutes

D. Every one to two hours

XXXXXDXXXXX

5. You are collecting meal trays and notice that your patient didn't eat much dinner. You should:

A. Remove the tray and record the amount eaten

B. Ask the patient if she would like a different meal

C. Heat the food up and bring it back for the patient to try again

D. Leave the tray there for a while and pick it up later

XXXXXBXXXXX

6. How often should fresh water and ice be passed to your patients?

A. Every day

B. Every two hours

C. Every eight hours

D. Every twelve hours

XXXXXCXXXXX

7. Your patient ate all of the main course and one side dish. He still has one side dish leftover and doesn't want it. When you record how much the patient ate, how much do you put?

A. 25%

B. 50%

C. 80%

D. 75%

XXXXXDXXXXX

8. You see that your patient is on a NAS diet. You know that this means:

A. There should be no added salt

B. He is diabetic and there should be no additional sugar

C. No additional sides for the patient; he is on a weight restriction

D. He is on a normal diet with no restrictions

XXXXXAXXXXX

9. Your patient is diagnosed with dehydration. What changes should be made in the amount of fluids she consumes?

A. Restrict the amount of fluids she consumes per hour

B. Assign a certain amount of fluids to be consumed with each meal

C. Offer your patient a drink more frequently than normal

D. Insert a feeding tube so fluids can be forced into the body until the patient is healthy again

XXXXXCXXXXX

10. You are assigned to help a patient eat dinner and notice that his beverages must be thickened. This is because:

A. Thin liquids can cause the patient to choke

B. Thickened liquids taste better

C. Thickened liquids are more nutritious

D. Thin liquids aren't appropriate to drink with dinner

XXXXXAXXXXX

11. Your diabetic patient asks for an evening snack. Because she is a diabetic, you know the best snack for her is:

A. Sour cream and onion chips

B. Almonds

C. Pudding

D. Blueberry muffin

XXXXXBXXXXX

12. You are assigned to take care of a patient with cancer who is being treated with chemotherapy. You know that her eating habits and appetite will:

A. Be similar to the other patients

B. Decrease

C. Increase

D. Cause her to always be thirsty

XXXXXBXXXXX

13. Which of the following is NOT appropriate when feeding a patient?

A. Placing a clothing protector over his shirt in case of spills

B. Feeding him in ten minutes so you have a chance to feed all of your patients

C. Frequently offering a drink

D. Feeding small bites

XXXXXBXXXXX

14. You are getting a new patient on the unit who has a PEG tube. You know that you won't need to feed this patient because:

A. Only the family is allowed

B. He is on hospice and refuses to eat

C. He will be fed by a nurse through the tube

D. He is pre-surgery and won't be allowed to eat

XXXXXCXXXXX

15. The nurse tells you that one of the patients on your assignment is NPO. This means:

A. She has behavioral problems

B. She is on suicide watch

C. She is on life support

D. She isn't allowed to have anything to eat or drink

XXXXXDXXXXX

COURSE # 4 - ADL - Rest & Sleep

Compared to the sleep habits of young adults, elderly adults need:

To take naps more often

Rationale: The elderly often have trouble sleeping during the night due to illness, stress, and hormonal changes such as decreased melatonin. This requires them to take naps throughout the day to re-energize them for activities.

Your patient rings her call light at midnight and tells you that she is having trouble sleeping. You should:

Notify the nurse

Rationale: Many patients have prescriptions or standing orders for a sleeping pill if they have difficulty sleeping. The nurse should be notified right away so the patient can be medicated early enough that the effects will have worn off by morning. Otherwise, the patient may not be able to accomplish her morning routine due to being groggy.

The following is something a nursing assistant can do to help a patient fall asleep:

Give a back rub

Rationale: A back rub is a simple task that a nursing assistant can do to help a patient fall asleep. Do not threaten the patient about still having to get up early. If the back rub doesn't work, a nurse can give the patient a sleeping pill, but passing out medications is not in the nursing assistant's scope of practice.

You are assigned to a patient who just had hip surgery. He rings his call light because he can't sleep. You know that this could be because:

He could be in pain from the surgery

Rationale: New post-op patients often have trouble resting and sleeping because they are in pain. Notify the nurse that the patient is having trouble sleeping and she may be able to treat the pain with medication. If that is unsuccessful, a sleeping pill may help.

The recommended number of hours of sleep an adult should get each night is:

Eight hours

Rationale: On average, adults should have eight hours of sleep at night to keep their bodies healthy and their minds functioning properly. Children may need up to eleven hours of sleep, and infants will sleep about sixteen hours a day.

----- COURSE TEST -----

1. Compared to the sleep habits of young adults, elderly adults need:

A. Less sleep

B. The same amount of sleep

C. To take naps more often

D. To sleep in later

XXXXXCXXXXX

2. Your patient rings her call light at midnight and tells you that she is having trouble sleeping. You should:

A. Fluff her pillow

B. Turn the TV on so she can have some background noise

C. Get her new bed sheets

D. Notify the nurse

XXXXXDXXXXX

3. Which of the following can a nursing assistant do to help a patient fall asleep?

A. Give a sleeping pill

B. Give a back rub

C. Hypnotize him

D. Threaten the patient that he will still have to get up early, even if he is tired

XXXXXBXXXXX

4. You are assigned to a patient who just had hip surgery. She rings her call light because she can't sleep, and you know that this could be because:

A. She is scared of the surgery

B. She is a night owl

C. She could be in pain from the surgery

D. The unit is too quiet

XXXXXCXXXXX

5. The recommended number of hours of sleep an adult should get each night is:

A. Eight hours

B. Ten hours

C. Six hours

D. Five hours

XXXXXAXXXXX

COURSE # 5 - Basic Skills - Data Collection & Reporting

The nurse asks you to take a patient's blood pressure. You notice that the blood pressure cuff is a bit too small. You should:

Find a blood pressure cuff that fits the patient

Rationale: A blood pressure cuff that is too small or too big can make the result inaccurate. A patient's treatment and blood pressure medications are adjusted according to the results, and inaccurate results can lead to unnecessary, and sometimes dangerous, changes. Always make sure the cuff fits appropriately according to the scale on the inside of the cuff.

You are bathing your patient and you notice a small abrasion on her wrist that you haven't noticed before. You should:

Notify the nurse of the abrasion after the bath

Rationale: Because the abrasion is on the wrist, the nurse can check it after the bath. If it is in a more discreet place like the buttocks, have another nursing assistant get the nurse. Never leave the patient alone while she is bathing. This is both a privacy and safety issue. Any skin issues that the nursing assistant thinks may be new should be brought to the attention of the nurse for evaluation and treatment.

The nurse should be notified of the following vital sign immediately:

Respirations of 28

Rationale: Respirations should be between twelve and twenty. When a patient is sleeping, this can be as low as eight to ten. If respirations are high, the patient is struggling to get enough air and is trying to breathe more rapidly to compensate. The nurse should be notified immediately because this patient may have an infection such as pneumonia and will need to be evaluated further.

The best time to do a skin assessment is:

While you are bathing the patient

Rationale: Doing a skin assessment while bathing the patient is the easiest and most efficient approach. Because the patient will already be undressed while being bathed, it is the best time to do a quick assessment for any new skin tears, bruises, abrasions, or reddened areas. It is unnecessary to undress the patient just to do a skin assessment because this takes away from her privacy. If there are any changes in the skin, notify the nurse.

You would NOT need to report the following to the nurse:

An Alzheimer's patient confused about what day it is

Rationale: In general, an Alzheimer's patient being confused about the day of the week isn't something abnormal. Only abnormal things should be reported to the nurse. If you are unsure as to whether it is normal or not, report it and let the nurse decide the next course of action.

You are taking a patient's pulse. You know that the normal pulse range is:

60-100 beats per minute

Rationale: A pulse of 60 to100 beats per minute is healthy. A pulse that is too high or too low isn't efficiently pumping blood to the rest of the body. Because oxygen is carried in the blood, the body isn't being properly oxygenated. This can cause problems in every body system. The nurse should be notified if the pulse is too high or too low.

The following location is the most common place for skin breakdown on a patient:

Coccyx

Rationale: The coccyx is the most common place for skin breakdown to occur and for ulcers to form. The most pressure is usually exerted on this area due to the patient's sitting and lying down. This area should be checked every day for changes, and any changes should be reported to the nurse. Pressure ulcers cost millions of dollars annually to treat. The earlier they're detected, the sooner the ulceration progression can be stopped.

A nursing assistant is allowed to do the following data collecting techniques:

Weighing the patient

Rationale: Part of a nursing assistant's job is to weigh patients and report any sudden changes to the nurse. All weights should be documented. Assessing a patient is not under the scope of practice for a nursing assistant, except checking the skin for new problems.

You are checking a patient's oxygen level with the pulse oximeter. It isn't reading well, and you notice the patient has fingernail polish on. Your next action would be:

Removing the nail polish on one finger and trying again

Rationale: Nail polish can interfere with the machine's ability to accurately determine a patient's oxygen level. Simply remove the nail polish on the finger you are using and trying again. This should fix the problem. If not, the machine may be broken and you should locate a new one.

The nurse asks you to check a patient's temperature orally. You know that you should never check a patient's temperature if:

She just finished drinking a beverage

Rationale: Drinking or eating right before having an oral temperature taken can make the results inaccurate. Instruct the patient not to eat or drink for fifteen minutes, and then return to the room and take the temperature. If the nursing assistant takes the temperature right after the patient has been eating or drinking, it may cause an incorrect reading. The patient may be unnecessarily treated if the food or drink was warm, or not treated when needed if the food or drink was cold.

You would report the following patient complaint to the nurse:

A patient claiming a nursing assistant is abusing her

Rationale: Any claims of abuse should be reported to the nurse immediately to be investigated. Even if the patient doesn't verbalize it and you suspect abuse or find bruises, you must still report it so it can be looked into further. Abuse is not only physical, but can also be sexual, mental, financial, or emotional.

You get ready to take a patient's blood pressure, knowing that a normal blood pressure is:

120/80 mmHg

Rationale: Blood pressure is the force that blood is exerting on the walls of the blood vessels. If it is too low or too high, it can be damaging to the body and have both short and long-term effects. There is a little bit of variation allowed, but anything below 100/50 or above 150/90 should be a concern and the nurse should be notified. Some patients have chronically low or high blood pressure and these can still be normal for that individual, but that is for the nurse to determine.

You should get a report about the patients you are assigned to:

At the beginning of your shift

Rationale: As a nursing assistant, you must ask your nurses for any information you may need to take care of your patients safely and effectively. This will include diagnosis, limitations, toileting habits, etc. You should always ask at the beginning of your shift because that is when you will start taking care of your patients, not in the middle of your shift or on a break.
Best practice guidelines are that the aide going off-duty will give you information on changes in conditions or problems that any patient is having. Some facilities require walking rounds to visualize the patients and make sure they are being left clean and dry. Other facilities see this practice as a potential privacy problem.

A nursing assistant is responsible for documenting which of the following:

Intake and output

Rationale: Nursing assistants are responsible for documenting a patient's intake and output, weight, mood, skin assessment, bathing, and toileting routines, as well as a number of other things. Nursing assistants are not allowed to perform physical assessments other than skin condition, nor do they give medications or treatments. Therefore, they will not document any information in those areas.

Knowing about the patients' conditions on the nursing assistant's shift assignment is the responsibility of:

The nursing assistant who will be working with those patients

Rationale: It is the responsibility of the nursing assistants to know about the conditions, treatments, etc., of the patients they care for. It is the CNA's responsibility to ask questions and read the Care Plan about each patient's toileting and bathing habits, ability to ambulate, and anything else related to the care the nursing assistant will provide. If a patient becomes injured because a nursing assistant did not get this information at the start of the shift, the nursing assistant can be held accountable in a court of law for negligence and can lose her job and license.

The following vital signs are abnormal and should be reported to the nurse immediately:

Oxygen saturation of 91%

Rationale: Normal oxygen saturation should be between 93% and 100%. Patients with chronic lung disease may have normal oxygen saturation as low as 85%, but anything lower than 93% should be reported to the nurse immediately so she can decide if it is normal for this patient's condition. If a patient is wearing oxygen, instruct him to breathe in through his nose and out through his mouth to improve his oxygen levels. Do not adjust the amount of oxygen he is receiving through the tank, even if the level is low.

Your patient fell earlier and you now notice a bruise on her thigh. You should:

Notify the nurse

Rationale: Injuries may not show up immediately after a patient falls. Any new injuries should be reported to the nurse right away. Assessing the patient for further injury is something the nurse will do when she checks on the bruised thigh.

When checking a pulse manually, you will check it:

On the wrist

Rationale: When manually checking a heart rate, check the radial pulse located on the patient's wrist. This will be on the palm side of the wrist, located below the thumb. Use your index and middle finger to do this, not the thumb. You can count the pulse for fifteen seconds and then multiply it by four. For the most accurate result, you should count for a full 60 seconds, especially if the heart rate is irregular.

It is important for the nursing assistant to document a patient's vital signs because:

The nurses and physicians can see if there are any changes from the patient's normal vitals

Rationale: The purpose of documentation is so that nurses and physicians can monitor any changes in a patient's condition. Without knowing the pattern of vital signs, they won't be able to tell if there is a variation from the patient's normal condition or not. Although a patient has a heart rate of 90, their normal could be 60. This drastic difference can only be noted if vital signs are documented consistently. Make sure that all vitals are documented by the end of your shift according to your employer's policy or the doctor's order for individual patients.

The following vital sign is abnormal and should be reported immediately:

Temperature of 100.7

Rationale: Anything above 100 degrees should be reported to the nurse for further evaluation. This is the first sign of an infection and it should be treated quickly.

----- COURSE TEST -----

1. The nurse asks you to take a patient's blood pressure. You notice that the blood pressure cuff is a bit too small. You should:

A. Continue to take the blood pressure

B. Take the blood pressure twice and average the two

C. Find a blood pressure cuff that fits the patient

D. Ask the patient if it feels too small and then decide what to do

XXXXXCXXXXX

2. You are bathing your patient and you notice a small abrasion on her wrist that you haven't noticed before. You should:

A. Notify the nurse of the abrasion after the bath

B. Leave the patient and get the nurse

C. Put a bandage on it after the bath

D. Monitor it to see if it heals, but if not, notify the nurse

XXXXXAXXXXX

3. Which of the following vital signs should the nurse be notified of immediately?

A. Blood pressure of 110/77

B. Respirations of 28

C. Pulse of 96

D. Temperature of 97.1

XXXXXBXXXXX

4. The best time to do a skin assessment is:

A. While the patient is in bed

B. Before the patient lies down

C. While you are bathing the patient

D. First thing in the morning

XXXXXCXXXXX

5. Which of the following would you NOT need to report to the nurse?

A. A patient complaining of elbow pain

B. A patient with a bloody nose

C. A patient complaining of nausea

D. An Alzheimer's patient confused about what day it is

XXXXXDXXXXX

6. You are taking a patient's pulse. You know that the normal pulse range is:

A. 75-100 beats per minute

B. 60-100 beats per minute

C. 50-75 beats per minute

D. 80-120 beats per minute

XXXXXBXXXXX

7. Which of the following locations is the most common place for skin breakdown on a patient?

A. Coccyx

B. Shoulder blade

C. Elbow

D. Knee

XXXXXAXXXXX

8. As a nursing assistant, you are allowed to do which of the following data collecting techniques?

A. Assessing the patient's lung sounds

B. Checking the patient's ankles for edema

C. Weighing the patient

D. Neurological assessment

XXXXXCXXXXX

9. You are checking a patient's oxygen level with the pulse oximeter. It isn't reading well, and you notice the patient has fingernail polish on. Your next action would be:

A. Removing the nail polish on one finger and trying again

B. Switching to another finger

C. Getting another machine

D. Changing the batteries of the machine

XXXXXAXXXXX

10. The nurse asks you to check a patient's temperature. You know that you should never check a patient's temperature if:

A. She is lying down

B. She just finished drinking a beverage

C. She is taking aspirin

D. She feels cold

XXXXXBXXXXX

11. You would report which of the following patient complaints to the nurse?

A. Temperature of 99.3

B. A patient not liking the curtains in his room

C. A patient claiming a nursing assistant is abusing him

D. A patient not liking the shirt he is wearing today

XXXXXCXXXXX

12. You get ready to take a patient's blood pressure, knowing that a normal blood pressure is:

A. 130/60 mmHg

B. 100/70 mmHg

C. 140/80 mmHg

D. 120/80 mmHg

XXXXXDXXXXX

13. When should you get a report about the patients you are assigned to?

A. At the beginning of your shift

B. During your first break

C. Before you go to lunch

D. The previous shift you work

XXXXXAXXXXX

14. A nursing assistant is responsible for documenting which of the following:

A. The wound treatments she performed

B. Intake and output

C. Where she gave insulin injections

D. How swollen a patient's ankles are

XXXXXBXXXXX

15. Whose responsibility is it to make sure that the nursing assistant knows about the care required for patients on his/her assignment?

A. The charge nurse

B. The nursing assistant on the previous shift

C. The director of nursing

D. The nursing assistant who will be working with those patients

XXXXXDXXXXX

16. Which of the following vital signs is abnormal and should be reported to the nurse immediately?

A. Blood pressure of 122/68 mmHg

B. Respirations of 14

C. Oxygen saturation of 91%

D. Pulse of 97

XXXXXCXXXXX

17. Your patient fell earlier and you now notice a bruise on her thigh. You should:

A. Notify the nurse

B. Do nothing, since bruises are expected after a patient falls

C. Only report it if the patient complains of pain

D. Assess the rest of the body for further injuries

XXXXXAXXXXX

18. When checking a pulse manually, you will check it:

A. On the forearm

B. On the foot

C. On the neck

D. On the wrist

XXXXXDXXXXX

19. It is important for the nursing assistant to document a patient's vital signs because:

A. The State Board of Nursing can sue if they aren't documented properly

B. The nurses and physicians can see if there are any changes from the patient's normal vitals

C. That's what the nurse tells you to do

D. Documentation is needed to prove a nursing assistant worked during the shift

XXXXXBXXXXX

20. The following vital sign is abnormal and should be reported immediately:

A. Blood pressure of 102/70

B. Pulse of 79

C. Temperature of 100.7

D. Respirations of 19

XXXXXCXXXXX

COURSE # 6 - Basic Skills - Infection Control

You are taking care of a patient suspected of having tuberculosis. The following type of protective equipment should be worn whenever you enter this patient's room:

Mask

Rationale: Tuberculosis is transmitted through droplets that come out of the infected patient's mouth and enter through the nose or mouth of a healthy person. By wearing a special filter mask, the infected droplets are prevented from entering the healthy person's body. Your employer will have a special type of filter mask for this situation, because a regular mask may not fully protect you.

You are assigned to a patient who has a diagnosis of Clostridium Difficile (C-Diff). He has diarrhea, and after changing his adult brief, the nursing assistant must:

Wash her hands to prevent the spread of infection

Rationale: C-Diff is spread because the spores from the infection are transferred and ingested. Fecal-oral transmission is how it is spread, which means spores on the hands are ingested through the mouth. Spores cannot be killed by simply using an alcohol based sanitizer. Hands must be washed with soap and warm water for thirty seconds. Gloves are worn during care for a patient with C-Diff, with proper hand hygiene before and after patient contact.

If you are accidentally stuck with a dirty needle, you should immediately:

Wash the area

Rationale: If you are stuck, first clean the wound with soap and warm water. Do not squeeze or pinch blood from the wound, or clean it with bleach. Wash the area for at least two minutes. When the wound is clean, you will then report the incident to the charge nurse, fill out the proper paperwork, and have blood drawn to test for hepatitis, HIV, and other blood borne diseases. Your doctor may prescribe antibiotics as a precaution. Typically, you will have blood work drawn again several months after the initial incident to retest for any diseases.

The quickest, cheapest, and easiest way to prevent the spread of infection is:

Hand washing

Rationale: Hand washing before and after contact with each patient has proven to be the best way to prevent the spread of infection between patients and employees. Using soap and warm water and washing the hands for thirty seconds is the most effective way to kill germs. Take special care under and around fingernails and between fingers. Using hand sanitizer is acceptable in most circumstances between hand washings, except when the patient has C-Diff, MRSA, or other infections that your facility deems hand sanitizer inappropriate.

It's necessary to take special precautions when you are taking care of a patient diagnosed with MRSA because:

MRSA is a serious infection that is hard to treat

Rationale: MRSA, or methicillin resistant staph aureus, is an infection that can't be treated by most antibiotics normally prescribed. It is resistant to their effects; therefore, a limited number of antibiotics will successfully treat it, and may not treat it in time to save a life. MRSA can continue to spread, eventually causing infection in the blood (sepsis) if it isn't treated quickly and with the right antibiotics.

You would use standard precautions with the following types of patients:

All patients

Rationale: Standard precautions should be used with all patients. Standard precautions are designed to prevent the spread of diseases and infections, even when you don't know they are present. These precautions include protective equipment like gloves and hand washing after each patient.

PPE stands for:

Personal protective equipment

Rationale: PPE, or personal protective equipment, is the primary barrier between you and a sick patient. It includes gloves, gowns, masks, shoe covers, respirators, face shields, safety glasses, and more. This equipment is specially designed to protect you from hazards like contaminated blood or sputum.

The following is NOT a blood borne pathogen:

RSV

Rationale: RSV is a respiratory virus that infects children and is not transmitted via the blood. Blood borne pathogens include HIV, Hepatitis B, and Hepatitis C. These are the most commonly known and can be spread through a single droplet of infected blood entering the body through an orifice, cut, or any open area.

While emptying a urine drainage bag, a splash of urine accidentally gets in your eye. The first thing to do is:

Flush your eye with water

Rationale: Infectious diseases can be transmitted through accidental exposure to the mucous membrane of the eye. If a patient's urine contains a bacteria or virus, you may be at risk. Any contact with the eye from urine, blood, or air-borne droplets, such as a cough or sneeze, should be considered infectious and treated immediately. Most healthcare settings are required to have an eye wash station to rinse the eye quickly and efficiently. If no eye wash station is available, rinse with lukewarm tap water for five minutes. Report the splash to the nurse and follow the protocol for completing paperwork and blood testing.

The following vaccine is offered to healthcare workers through their place of employment:

Hepatitis B

Rationale: Healthcare workers are offered Hepatitis B vaccines by their employers to prevent the contraction and spread of this disease. It is not required, but highly recommended. It is a series of three shots. The first shot can be given anytime, the second shot is given one month after the first injection, and the third is given six months after the first dose. It is very safe and has very few potential side effects.

The following is NOT a requirement for a sharps container:

Red in color

Rationale: The color of the container doesn't affect its safety, but it must have a biohazard label on it. It should also be puncture resistant, closable, and leak proof. There are proper ways to dispose of these containers, and your employer will have more information about their policies. Biohazard containers do not go in a normal wastebasket or garbage can.

An inappropriate place to wear personal protective equipment would be:

The cafeteria

Rationale: Personal protective equipment should only be worn in patient environments where you have a chance of being exposed to body fluids and blood borne pathogens. A cafeteria is a "clean area" and should not be contaminated with personal protective equipment. Common hospital areas, such as the cafeteria, are used by hospital employees and visitors. It is important to keep these areas safe for everyone.

You are accidentally stuck with a dirty needle. You should report the incident immediately because:

Blood work needs to be drawn

Rationale: Regardless of whether you think the needle was contaminated, you should report it immediately. Your blood will be tested for possible infection, including hepatitis, HIV, and other blood borne diseases. This blood test is for your own safety and protection.

A healthcare worker should get a PPD test for tuberculosis:

Every year

Rationale: Healthcare workers are usually required by their facility to get a PPD test annually. It consists of a very small injection into one of the forearms. It is assessed two to three days later to see if there is a reaction or not. A positive PPD test does not necessarily mean you have tuberculosis. A chest x-ray and sputum culture must be taken to officially diagnose the disease.

You accidentally spill body fluids on the outside of a biohazard bag. You should:

Place that bag inside of another biohazard bag

Rationale: All body fluids must be contained in a biohazard container to prevent the chance of contracting a blood borne pathogen. If the outside of the container is contaminated, simply place it inside of another one. Do not throw it away in a regular wastebasket, or leave it for someone else to clean up.

----- COURSE TEST -----

1. You are taking care of a patient suspected of having tuberculosis. What type of protective equipment should be worn whenever you enter this patient's room?

A. Gown

B. Gloves

C. Mask

D. Shoe covers

XXXXXCXXXXX

2. You are assigned to a patient who has a diagnosis of Clostridium Difficile (C-Diff). He has diarrhea, and after changing the adult brief, the nursing assistant must:

A. Use hand sanitizer to prevent the spread of infection

B. Wash her hands to prevent the spread of infection

C. Inform the nurse of the diarrhea

D. Answer the call lights that rang while you were with that patient

XXXXXBXXXXX

3. If you are accidently stuck with a dirty needle, you should immediately:

A. Wash the area

B. Get tested for diseases such as HIV and hepatitis

C. Report it to your supervisor

D. Fill out an incident report

XXXXXAXXXXX

4. What is the quickest, cheapest, and easiest way to prevent the spread of infection?

A. Hand washing

B. Yearly testing for C-Diff for both patients and employees

C. Starting both patients and employees on antibiotics at the first sign of infection

D. Sterilizing all shared equipment, such as blood pressure cuffs and wheelchairs

XXXXXAXXXXX

5. It is necessary to take special precautions when you are taking care of a patient diagnosed with MRSA because:

A. It is transmitted through droplets and a mask should be worn

B. MRSA is a flesh-eating virus

C. MRSA will always be in your body if you are exposed to it

D. MRSA can be a serious infection and is hard to treat

XXXXXDXXXXX

6. What type of patient would you use standard precautions with?

A. A patient with open wounds

B. A patient with diarrhea

C. A patient having a heart attack

D. All patients

XXXXXDXXXXX

7. PPE stands for:

A. People protection environment

B. Personal protective equipment

C. Personal prevention equipment

D. Parasite protection equipment

XXXXXBXXXXX

8. Which of the following is NOT a blood borne pathogen?

A. HIV

B. RSV

C. Hepatitis C

D. Hepatitis B

XXXXXBXXXXX

9. While emptying a urine drainage bag, a splash of urine accidentally get in your eye. What should you do first?

A.   Flush your eye with water

B.   Check the patient's chart for the most recent urinalysis

C.   Ask the nurse for antibiotic eye drops

D.   Wash your hands after emptying the bag

XXXXXAXXXXX

10. Vaccines for which of the following diseases are offered to the healthcare worker through his place of employment?

A. Hepatitis A

B. HIV

C. Hepatitis B

D. AIDS

XXXXXCXXXXX

11. Which of the following is NOT a requirement for a sharps container?

A. Red in color

B. Puncture resistant

C. Closable

D. Labeled

XXXXXAXXXXX

12. An inappropriate place to wear personal protective equipment would be:

A. The laboratory

B. A trauma room

C. The cafeteria

D. In surgery

XXXXXCXXXXX

13. You are accidentally stuck with a dirty needle. You should report the incident immediately because:

A. A physician's note is required to continue work

B. Quality Assurance must be notified

C. The sharps container box should be changed

D. Blood work needs to be drawn for testing

XXXXXDXXXXX

14. How often should a healthcare worker get a PPD test to check for tuberculosis?

A. Every two years

B. Every six months

C. Every year

D. Every five years

XXXXXCXXXXX

15. You accidentally spill body fluids on the outside of a biohazard bag. You should:

A. Place that bag inside of another biohazard bag

B. Throw it in the trashcan immediately

C. Set it in the dirty utility room for housekeeping to clean up

D. Leave it—biohazard bags are made to soak in body fluids in case of spills

XXXXXAXXXXX

COURSE # 7 - Basic Skills - Fall Prevention

You enter a patient's room and find that she has fallen on the floor. You immediately:

Have someone get the nurse

Rationale: If you find a patient who has fallen, do not leave her. Yell for someone to get the nurse immediately. Do not move the patient, because she may be injured and moving her can worsen the injury. The nurse must assess the patient before she can be moved.

The following percentages of adults over the age of 65 have a chance of falling:

33%

Rationale: One in three adults over 65 will fall. Falls increase the chance of injury, which can lead to an early death, especially in patients who fracture a hip.

The following will NOT help in preventing falls:

Placing throw rugs around the patient's room so he can get traction while walking

Rationale: Loose rugs can dramatically increase a patient's chance of tripping and falling. They should be removed from any areas that the patient walks. Making sure the room is well-lit and clutter-free is important. People over 65 should have their hearing and vision checked yearly.

The doctor writes a prescription for your patient to have a pressure alarm. The purpose of this type of alarm is:

To prevent falls

Rationale: Pressure alarms work by alarming only when pressure is taken off of the pad because a patient is trying to stand or walk. Nursing assistants should respond immediately to these alarms in order to prevent injury from a fall.

A safety issue for a patient with a history of falls would include:

No hand rails in the shower

Rationale: Patients with fall risks should have as many adaptations as possible to prevent a fall. Having a handrail in the shower will help the patient stabilize herself while she showers. Other adaptations include using a walker while ambulating, using a raised toilet seat, and getting a bed that can be lowered to the floor each night.

As a CNA, you will fill out this type of paperwork after you find a patient who has fallen:

Witness statement

Rationale: After a fall, there are several forms that must be filled out. The nurse will take care of most of the forms, but if you are the nursing assistant who found the patient, you must fill out a witness statement accurately describing how and where you found the patient.

If a patient has an order to have an alarm on, it should be on:

At all times

Rationale: Alarms prevent falls. Since falls can occur at any time, alarms should always be on and attached to the patient. This includes during sleep, meals, and when in a wheelchair, if applicable. Not attaching the alarm to the patient is negligence. A nursing assistant could lose her job over this, especially if injury occurs.

After a fall, patients usually fracture a bone because of:

Osteoporosis

Rationale: Osteoporosis is the thinning of bone tissue and a loss of bone density that occurs with age. Bones aren't able to tolerate as much trauma with this disease, so a fall can fracture one or multiple bones at the same time. This costs thousands of dollars to fix and heal, including a long stay in the hospital and in rehabilitation.

You are walking with a patient and he starts to fall. The best thing to do next is:

Slide him down your leg onto the ground

Rationale: If a patient is falling, don't forcefully try to prevent the fall. This can injure joints or cause skin tears. Simply lean the patient into you and slide him down your leg to cause minimum impact on the ground. Then stay with the patient and have someone go get the nurse to assess the patient.

You are taking care of a confused patient who is a fall risk and keeps trying to stand up. The following is an appropriate way to try to prevent falling:

Distract him by turning on his favorite TV show

Rationale: A confused patient can often be distracted by giving him something to do, such as turning on his favorite show. Restraining him is not allowed without a doctor's order, and is something only a nurse can do. He should never be left alone, because he is more likely to try and stand up on his own and fall.

1. You enter a patient's room and find that she has fallen on the floor. You immediately:

A. Help her up

B. Have someone get the nurse

C. Roll her to her side

D. Leave her and go get the nurse

XXXXXBXXXXX

2. What percentage of adults over the age of 65 has a chance of falling?

A. 61%

B. 20%

C. 33%

D. 47%

XXXXXCXXXXX

3. Which of the following will NOT help prevent falls?

A. Placing throw rugs around the patient's room so she can get traction while walking

B. Making sure the room is well lit

C. Removing clutter from areas where the patient walks

D. Having the patient's hearing and vision checked every year

XXXXXAXXXXX

4. The doctor writes a prescription for your patient to have a pressure alarm. What is the purpose of an alarm?

A. To notify the nurse of weight loss

B. To prevent skin breakdown from pressure on the buttocks

C. To prevent falls

D. To notify the nurse that the patient is ambulating

XXXXXCXXXXX

5. Which of the following would be a safety issue for a patient with a history of falls?

A. Using a walker

B. A raised toilet seat in the bathroom

C. Low bed height

D. No hand rails in the shower

XXXXXDXXXXX

6. What type of paperwork will you need to fill out after you find a patient who has fallen?

A. Workers compensation paper

B. Incident report

C. Witness statement

D. Ambulance transfer papers

XXXXXCXXXXX

7. If a patient has an order to have an alarm on, when should it be on?

A. At all times

B. While in bed

C. While in a wheelchair

D. While walking

XXXXXAXXXXX

8. After a fall, patients usually fracture a bone because of what disease?

A. Cancer

B. Osteoporosis

C. Diabetes

D. CHF

XXXXXBXXXXX

9. You are walking with a patient and she starts to fall. What is the best thing to do next?

A. Lean her toward you and slide her down your leg onto the ground

B. Shout for help as she is falling

C. Hold onto whatever you can to prevent the fall

D. Let her fall onto you

XXXXXAXXXXX

10. You are taking care of a confused patient who is a fall risk and keeps trying to stand up. Which of the following is an appropriate way to try to prevent falling?

A. Restrain her to the wheelchair

B. Put her to bed

C. Distract her by turning on her favorite TV show

D. Leave her alone so she stops trying to get attention

XXXXXCXXXXX

COURSE # 8 - Basic Skills - Medical Emergencies

You find your patient unresponsive and not breathing. You should immediately:

Shout for help

Rationale: An unresponsive patient should never be left alone. Shout for help immediately. The nurse will respond to the patient and begin CPR if the patient's Living Will allows her to do so.

You notice your patient is having trouble speaking and he isn't able to use his left arm very well. You notify the nurse immediately because your patient may be having:

A stroke

Rationale: Signs of a stroke include trouble speaking, weakness on one side of the body, facial drooping, confusion, and trouble seeing. Any of these signs should be reported to the nurse immediately for evaluation. The longer a stroke goes untreated, the more damage there is. If a stroke can be treated within 90 minutes, the patient has a very good chance of not having any permanent deficits.

You would immediately notify the nurse of:

A pulse of 41

Rationale: A pulse of 41 is low. Normal pulse rate should be between 60 and 100 beats per minute. When the pulse (heart rate) is too slow, not enough blood is being perfused throughout the body. Because oxygen travels in the blood, the body may not be getting enough oxygen. Although this low heart rate may be normal for some patients, it is for the nurse to decide if it normal, so she should be notified immediately.

CNAs should renew their CPR cards every:

Two years

Rationale: Because a CNA may play a part in performing CPR on a patient who is in cardiac arrest, she must renew her CPR card every two years. The sooner CPR is performed on a patient having a heart attack, the better chance that patient has of living without any permanent damage. Many facilities require that you have your CPR card and will pay for you to take the class in order to keep your card up to date.

The following is considered a medical emergency:

Blood in the stool

Rationale: Blood in the stool signifies that the patient is bleeding somewhere. Although the bleeding could just be from a hemorrhoid, the patient should be checked by a physician to make sure the bleeding is not life threatening. If you have a patient with blood in her stool, notify the nurse immediately. Do not flush or dispose of the stool because the nurse will need to assess it.

Your patient rings his call light and tells you that his chest hurts. Your first action is to:

Notify the nurse immediately

Rationale: Chest pain can be a sign of a something serious like a heart attack, or something benign like heart burn. The CNA should notify the nurse of the patient's complaint so the nurse can access him and take further action. The CNA is not allowed to assess the patient or begin treatment. Even if the CNA thinks it is nothing, she must notify the nurse of the patient's complaint.

You notice that your patient's urine has been darker and has a foul odor. You notify the nurse of this change because it is a sign of:

Urinary tract infection

Rationale: Sign of a UTI are burning during urination, dark urine, frequent urges to urinate, and foul smelling urine. If left untreated, a UTI can turn into a kidney infection, or even kidney failure. In older patients, UTIs can cause confusion and disorientation. If you have an older patient who seems confused or disoriented, check the urine for any changes and report them to the nurse.

You enter a patient's room and find him not breathing. He has a DNR order. This means that you should now do which of the following:

Call for the nurse, but do not start CPR

Rationale: When a patient or family member signs a DNR, this means no extraordinary measures are to be taken to save the patient in case of severe illness or death. It is the nurse's ultimate decision and knowledge to decide whether or not CPR is to be performed, but if there is a signed and legal DNR, CPR is not performed. Call for the nurse immediately. She will decide the next course of action.

If you discover a fire, you should R,A.C.E. R:A.C.E. stands for:

Rescue, alarm, contain, evacuate

Rationale: According to OSHA fire safety, R.A.C.E. is the acronym that should be followed in case of a fire. Rescue any patients in the vicinity of the fire who could be in immediate danger (without injuring yourself), alarm the building, contain the fire by closing doors and windows, and evacuate the building of all patients, employees, and visitors.

You are assigned to a patient who has a history of seizures. As a nursing assistant, you are most concerned about the patient's:

Safety

Rationale: The nursing assistant should be constantly aware of the safety of any patient, but especially for one with a history of seizures. Look around the room for anything that could be dangerous if a patient begins to seize, and make sure the side rails of the bed are padded as allowed by your facility. It is the responsibility of all employees to make sure every patient is safe, but as a nursing assistant, this will be your priority with this type of patient.

You are assigned to a patient who has lost a lot of blood due to a tear in his intestine. He is receiving blood for the first time. When changing him, you notice he has a new rash. You notify the nurse immediately because he:

Could be having a reaction to the blood he is receiving

Rationale: Although most patients don't have reactions to receiving blood, it does occur. The nurse will stay with the patient and monitor him for several minutes initially to make sure nothing negative occurs. A rash is one of the first signs that the body is having a reaction to something. If the patient is reacting to the blood, it could have deadly results.

Your patient is a diabetic and tells you that she thinks her sugar is getting low. You should:

Notify the nurse

Rationale: Diabetic patients often can sense when their blood sugar isn't right. The nursing assistant should immediately notify the nurse so she can delegate a further course of action. Some nursing assistants are allowed to check a patient's blood sugar. This will be the first step. The nurse may then ask you to get the patient some orange juice to raise her blood sugar if it is low. No steps should be taken by the nursing assistant without the approval of the nurse.

While bathing a patient, she tells you she is going to take all of her medication today because she just wants to die. You react by:

Having someone else notify the nurse while you stay with the patient

Rationale: Whenever a patient threatens to harm herself, she should never be left alone. The nurse should be notified immediately so she can further assess the patient. No matter how small the threat may be, it should always be taken seriously. The nursing assistant isn't allowed to remove the patient's medications or dispose of them, so just stay with the patient until you are given further instructions by the nurse.

While you are taking vital signs on a patient, you notice the patient's pulse is jumping from 90 to 120 beats per minute on the machine you're using. Your next action should be:

To manually check the patient's pulse

Rationale: Because machines can malfunction, the nursing assistant should manually check the pulse before reporting it to the nurse. There are certain heart conditions where the pulse can jump erratically, but these can only be determined by a physician. If the manual re-check is similar to what the machine said, notify the nurse immediately.

You are taking care of a patient who hasn't voided at all during your twelve hour shift. You notify the nurse, knowing that the next step is:

Inserting a catheter

Rationale: Urinating is the body's way of removing toxins. If these toxins aren't removed, they are harmful to the patient. An average of 30ml per hour is normal urine output. No output for twelve hours is something that should be dealt with immediately. CNAs generally aren't allowed to insert a catheter, but often assist the nurse with the procedure. Inserting a catheter will show whether the patient is unable to begin the urination process, or if she is not making any urine. Both should be treated urgently.

----- COURSE TEST -----

1. You find your patient unresponsive and not breathing. You should immediately:

A. Shout for help

B. Move the patient to the floor

C. Give two rescue breaths

D. Leave the room and find someone to help you

XXXXXAXXXXX

2. You notice your patient is having trouble speaking and he isn't able to use his left arm very well. You notify the nurse immediately because your patient may be having:

A. A heart attack

B. A stroke

C. A seizure

D. A septic episode

XXXXXBXXXXX

3. Which of the following would you notify the nurse of immediately?

A. Blood pressure of 130/95

B. Temperature of 99.2

C. Oxygen saturation of 93%

D. A pulse of 41

XXXXXDXXXXX

4. CNAs should renew their CPR cards every:

A. Two years

B. Five years

C. Six months

D. One year

XXXXXAXXXXX

5. Which of the following is considered a medical emergency?

A. Diarrhea

B. Vomiting

C. Blood in stool

D. Gout

XXXXXCXXXXX

6. Your patient rings his call light and tells you that his chest hurts. Your first action is to:

A. Tell him it's because he is tired and should get some sleep

B. Ask him to point to where it hurts

C. Give him one of the Tylenol you have for your headaches

D. Notify the nurse immediately

XXXXXDXXXXX

7. You notice that your patient's urine has become darker and has a foul odor. You notify the nurse of this change because it is a sign of:

A. Pancreatitis

B. Urinary tract infection

C. Appendicitis

D. Diabetes

XXXXXBXXXXX

8. You enter a patient's room to find her not breathing. She has a DNR. This means that you should now do which of the following:

A. Call for the nurse, but do not start CPR

B. Call for the nurse and immediately start CPR

C. Give two rescue breaths and then call for the nurse if the patient doesn't start breathing

D. Begin CPR and have another nursing assistant perform mouth to mouth

XXXXXAXXXXX

9. If you discover a fire, you should R.A.C.E. What does R.A.C.E. stand for?

A. Rescue, alarm, contain, evacuate

B. Rescue, alarm, commit, evaluate

C. Remove, alert, confine, and elope

D. Remove, alarm, contain, evaluate

XXXXXAXXXXX

10. You are assigned to a patient who has a history of seizures. As a nursing assistant, you are most concerned about the patient's:

A. Medication regimen

B. Airway

C. Safety

D. IV

XXXXXCXXXXX

11. You are assigned to a patient who has lost a lot of blood due to a tear in his intestine. He is receiving blood for the first time. When changing him, you notice he has a new rash. You notify the nurse immediately because he:

A. May be bleeding internally again

B. Must be allergic to the bed sheets

C. Is itching too much and irritating his skin

D. Could be having a reaction to the blood he is receiving

XXXXXDXXXXX

12. Your patient is a diabetic and tells you that she thinks her sugar is getting low. You should:

A. Get her a glass of orange juice

B. Inject her with insulin

C. Check her blood sugar

D. Notify the nurse

XXXXXDXXXXX

13. While bathing a patient, she tells you she is going to take all of her medication today because she just wants to die. You react by:

A. Leaving her alone to finish bathing herself

B. Having someone else notify the nurse while you stay with the patient

C. Throwing her medicine away

D. Notifying the nurse of the patient's threats

XXXXXBXXXXX

14. While taking vital signs on a patient, you notice the patient's pulse is jumping from 90 to 120 beats per minute on the machine you're using. Your next action should be:

A. To disregard the reading because the machine must be broken

B. To manually check the patient's pulse

C. To notify the nurse of the results

D. Have the patient stand up and re-check the pulse

XXXXXBXXXXX

15. You are taking care of a patient who hasn't voided at all during your twelve hour shift. You notify the nurse, knowing that the next step is:

A. Insert a catheter

B. Order a CT scan

C. Help the patient to the bedside commode

D. Have the next shift monitor the patient

XXXXXAXXXXX

COURSE # 9 - Behavior and Mental Health

You notice that your resident is less social than normal and tends to want to stay in bed all day. You notify the nurse because these are signs of:

Depression

Rationale: Although depression is believed by many to just be part of the aging process, it is something that needs to be treated and dealt with just like any other disease. Signs of depression include changes in sleep habits, changes in eating habits, changes in mood, trouble concentrating, or feeling worthless or sad.

You are taking care of a very angry patient who was just admitted to your facility. You should help the patient deal with his anger by:

Letting the patient discuss his feelings with you

Rationale: Talking out a patient's feelings and listening to him discuss things is the best way you can help an angry patient feel better. Don't antagonize him or threaten him, as this can make the situation worse. If you are concerned that the patient may become violent, let the nurse know so that the safety of the other patients and staff isn't compromised.

You are taking care of an Alzheimer's patient who is very confused. The following is an inappropriate way to deal with this type of patient:

Explaining everything with great detail until it is understood

Rationale: When dealing with someone who is confused, use short, simple sentences to get your point across. The more detailed and lengthy your sentences are, the more confused the patient may become. Keep it simple!

The following is NOT a factor that can cause depression in a patient:

The birth of a grandchild

Rationale: Depression can be caused by many things, including the loss of friends or family, a change in sleep habits or nutrition, a new lifestyle, or being diagnosed with a new disease. If you suspect your patient might be depressed, notify the nurse so she can speak with the patient about it and alert the doctor.

Your patient told you that when his roommate is angry, he tries to hit him. The first thing you should do is:

Remove the non-violent patient

Rationale: Although it is rare, roommate conflict does occur. Safety of the patients should be everyone's biggest concern. First, remove the patient who is being hit. Then, notify the nurse of the situation. She can take the next steps in providing a safe environment for both patients.

The following statement is true regarding mental health in the elderly:

Psychosis is considered a mental health disorder

Rationale: Mental health concerns specific to the elderly include dementia, delirium, psychosis, and depression. One-third of patients diagnosed with mental health disorders are untreated. If you are concerned your patient may have a change in mental status, notify the nurse so she can assess the patient and investigate further.

The following is something nursing assistants are allowed to do when they are taking care of a violent patient:

Move the patient to a private area and speak with her

Rationale: Unless there is a physician's order in place, restraints can never be placed regardless of whether they are physical or medicinal. Threatening a patient may only agitate him more and cause the situation to escalate. Allowing the patient to vent his feelings may make him feel more in control and relaxed.

The following is not a sign of depression:

Too much energy

Rationale: Changes in a person's sleeping and eating habits, as well as feelings of worthlessness and loss of interest in activities, are all signs of depression. Patients tend to have less energy, not more, when suffering from depression. If you notice any of these changes in your patient, notify the nurse.

A patient tells you she has been thinking about hurting herself because she is depressed. You should:

Stay with the patient and have someone get the nurse

Rationale: Never leave a patient alone if she is thinking of self-harm. Get another employee's attention and have him inform the nurse of the situation. Do not judge or yell at the patient. Only listen to her and be sympathetic to the situation.

You are taking care of a confused patient who is a fall risk and keeps trying to get out of his wheelchair. You should:

Place the patient in a well-monitored area

Rationale: Never leave a confused patient who is at risk for falling. Make sure he is somewhere in the facility or on the unit where he can be monitored by staff. The only exception to this is if he is in bed sleeping. Don't force the patient to go to bed if he is clearly awake. It may agitate him and make things worse.

----- COURSE TEST -----

1. You notice that your resident is less social than normal and tends to want to stay in bed all day. You notify the nurse because these are signs of:

A. Cancer

B. Psychotic disorder

C. Bipolar disorder

D. Depression

XXXXXDXXXXX

2. You are taking care of a very angry patient who was just admitted to your facility. You should help the patient deal with his anger by:

A. Allowing the patient to discuss his feelings with you

B. Telling him he will be moved to another facility if he becomes violent

C. Informing him that he will be heavily medicated unless his anger goes away

D. Not allowing family members to see him until he is happy again

XXXXXAXXXXX

3. You are taking care of an Alzheimer's patient who is very confused. The following is an inappropriate way to deal with this type of patient:

A. Redirecting the patient

B. Explaining everything with great detail until it is understood

C. Giving the patient a task that will occupy her time, such as setting the dinner tables

D. Taking the patient to participate in an activity

XXXXXBXXXXX

4. Which of the following is NOT a factor that can cause depression in a patient?

A. Loss of friends or family

B. The birth of a grandchild

C. Being diagnosed with a new disease

D. Lack of sleep

XXXXXBXXXXX

5. Your patient told you that when his roommate is angry, he tries to hit him. The first thing you should do is:

A. Remove the violent patient

B. Notify the nurse

C. Remove the non-violent patient

D. Inform the violent patient why actions are inappropriate

XXXXXCXXXXX

6. The following statement is true regarding mental health in the elderly:

A. Alzheimer's is the most common type of dementia

B. One in four women is at risk for depression

C. Age plays a large role in a patient's mental health status

D. Psychosis is considered a mental health disorder

XXXXXDXXXXX

7. Which of the following are nursing assistants allowed to do when they are taking care of a violent patient?

A. Move the patient to a private area and speak with him

B. Place restraints on the patient's arms so he cannot hit

C. Inform the patient that what he is doing is illegal and it can be punished by law

D. Give the patient medication to calm him down

XXXXXAXXXXX

8. Which of the following is not a sign of depression?

A. Change in eating habits

B. Change in sleeping habits

C. Too much energy

D. Loss of interest in social activities

XXXXXCXXXXX

9. A patient tells you she has been thinking about hurting herself because she is depressed. You should:

A. Get the nurse immediately

B. Stay with the patient and have someone get the nurse

C. Listen to the patient and then check back on her later

D. Call the patient's family to come in and cheer her up

XXXXXBXXXXX

10. You are taking care of a confused patient who is a fall risk and keeps trying to get out of his wheelchair. You should:

A. Place the patient in a well-monitored area

B. Take the patient to his room and turn on the TV

C. Lay the patient in bed, even if he isn't tired

D. Restrain him in his chair to prevent falling

XXXXXAXXXXX

COURSE # 10 - Blood Glucose Monitoring

Your patient is to have her blood glucose level monitored every morning. You will obtain this by:

A finger stick to obtain a drop of blood placed on a blood glucose monitor (glucometer)

Rationale: A blood glucose (sugar) level is typically obtained by a finger stick. This may be requested numerous times throughout the day for a patient, depending on the doctor's order. It is most often ordered in the morning, at night, and before or after meals. There are certain circumstances when blood sugar may be obtained when other labs are drawn, or if the patient has some type of IV access and the nurse is able to obtain the specimen. A blood glucose level is obtained by pricking the patient's finger with an approved single-use lancet, obtaining a drop of blood to place on the glucometer, and obtaining a reading. After use, the lancets should be disposed of in a sharps container.

Blood sugar levels are often requested on patients with this condition:

Diabetes

Rationale: Diabetes is a chronic condition in which the body has a problem with making insulin, producing the correct amount of insulin to maintain healthy glucose levels, or insulin resistance. Diabetic patients require frequent checks of their blood sugar to guide their therapy and treatment. Blood glucose monitoring reveals individual patterns of blood glucose changes. It is necessary for planning of meals, activities, and at what time of day to take medications.

When you are performing a blood glucose check on your patient and you are unable to obtain a full drop of blood for testing, you should:

Lower the hand below the level of the waist, wrap the hand with a warm cloth, and try again in five minutes

Rationale: Certain factors can make it difficult to obtain a full drop of blood for a blood glucose level. It is helpful to warm the fingers and to lower the hand below the waist to increase the blood flow to the fingers. It is important that accurate blood levels are recorded. It is never acceptable to record what the blood glucose "usually" runs.

Your blood glucometer is out of testing strips. When replacing the strips from the supply closet, you should:

Match the new test strips to the glucometer and program, as directed

Rationale: Blood glucometers come with specific test strips which are identified by batch number. The number of the test strip must match the number that the glucometer is set for. This is to be done anytime you begin using a new batch of test strips. Note that test strips expire, and only non-expired strips should be used. Testing strips may only be used one time and then disposed of as hazardous waste.

The CNA should prep the patient's finger by:

Cleaning it with an alcohol pad

Rationale: The finger should be cleansed with a 70% alcohol pad/solution, and the site should be allowed to dry completely before sticking the skin for a specimen. If you do not allow the site to dry completely, it could cause the blood to be contaminated, as well as increase pain for the patient. It is important to protect the patient and yourself from any exchange of bacteria or infection. The CNA should wear gloves, but other protective barriers such as eye shields or gowns are not necessary, as spurting blood is not a reasonable concern.

You check on your patient and find her to be sleepy and difficult to arouse. You inform the nurse and she asks for a blood glucose check on the patient. The glucose level is 29. You should:

Inform the nurse, as this is an emergency situation

Rationale: A normal glucose level range is between 80 and 120. A number lower than this is called hypoglycemia and can be a medical emergency. The nurse should be alerted immediately of this situation. Never wait or delay passing on information about a critical blood glucose level. Never attempt to feed a patient who is lethargic, as she is at a high risk of choking or aspirating whatever is put into the mouth. Also, do not attempt to get a patient out of bed who is lethargic or sleepy, as there would be an increased fall or accident risk.

Your patient has a blood sugar of 450. You should:

Inform the nurse of the high level

Rationale: High blood sugar is called hyperglycemia. The normal glucose range for a patient is 80 to 120. It is important to notify the nurse any time that the blood glucose level is not within the normal range. Delaying treatment of hypoglycemia or hyperglycemia can cause further medical problems for the patient.

When using a shared glucose meter in a long-term care facility, it is recommended to be cleaned:

After each patient

Rationale: Glucometers should be cleaned and disinfected after each patient to prevent the transmission of blood and infectious agents to the next patient. The guidelines for cleaning may differ slightly according to manufacturer, but the solution used must be effective against HIV, Hepatitis B, and Hepatitis C.

When you are performing any procedure and there is a potential exposure to blood or body fluids, you should:

Wear gloves

Rationale: You should always wear gloves when there is potential to come into contact with blood or body fluids. This is to protect you and the patient from transmission of bacteria and disease. Hands should always be washed before and after contact with a patient, even if gloves are worn. The CNA should wear gloves, but other protective barriers such as eye shields or a gown are not necessary, as spurting blood is not a reasonable concern.

The factor determining how often a diabetic patient's blood sugar should be tested is:

As indicated per doctor's order

Rationale: The amount of times that blood sugar levels are tested will vary per patient. There are numerous factors that will impact blood glucose levels, such as activity, medications, food intake, and health history. Some patients may have glucose levels checked once per day, while testing others' levels may be ordered several times per day. The nurse will indicate how frequently blood sugar testing needs to be completed on a patient each day. It is the responsibility of the CNA to report the results back to the nurse.

----- COURSE TEST -----

1. How do you obtain a patient's blood glucose level?

A. By weighing him

B. Obtain a urine specimen

C. A finger stick

D.   A stool specimen

XXXXXCXXXXX

2. What medical condition requires that blood sugar levels be taken on patients?

A. Diabetes

B. Urinary tract infections

C. Influenza

D. Chest pain

XXXXXAXXXXX

3. What should you do when you are performing a blood glucose check on your patient and you are unable to obtain a full drop of blood for testing?

A. Run the patient's hand under cold water

B. Raise the patient's hand into the air

C. Write down what the patient says their glucose "usually" runs

D. Lower the hand and wrap with a warm cloth and try again in five minutes

XXXXXDXXXXX

4. What should you do when you are replacing the strips for a blood glucometer from the supply closet?

A. Use any glucose strips that are in the supply room

B. Match the new test strips to the glucometer and program, as directed

C. Dispose of the glucometer

D. Reuse your last testing strip until someone replaces them

XXXXXBXXXXX

5. How should a CNA prep the patient's finger for a finger stick?

A. By blowing on it

B. By placing a latex glove on the patient's hand

C. By dipping it in water

D. By cleaning it with an alcohol pad

XXXXXDXXXXX

6. What should you do when you have been asked by a nurse to perform a finger stick glucose test on your patient who seems to be sleepy and difficult to arouse, and has a glucose level of 29?

A. Have the patient drink some juice

B. Inform the nurse, as this is an emergency situation

C. Get the patient out of bed to walk around

D. Recheck the blood sugar in two hours to see if it is the same result

XXXXXBXXXXX

7. What should you do when your patient has a blood sugar of 450?

A. Do nothing, as this is a normal blood glucose level

B. Inform the nurse of the high level

C. Get her some orange juice

D. Have the patient walk around to lower her glucose level

XXXXXBXXXXX

8. How often should you clean a shared glucose meter in a long-term care facility?

A. At the end of each shift

B. After each patient

C. Once a day

D. Once a week

XXXXXBXXXXX

9. What should you do when you are performing any procedure and there is a potential exposure to blood or body fluids?

A. Wear gloves

B. Refuse to perform the procedure

C. Ask someone else to do it

D. Wear an eye shield

XXXXXAXXXXX

10. How frequently should blood sugar levels be tested on a diabetic patient?

A. Once per week

B. Every hour

C. As indicated per doctor's order

D. Whenever the patient requests to have his level checked

XXXXXCXXXXX

COURSE # 11 - Client Rights

The purpose of the Patient's Bill of Rights is:

To teach patients the importance of a healthy and open patient-doctor relationship

Rationale: The Patient's Bill of Rights was created to help patients feel more confident in their physicians and in the healthcare system. The Patient's Bill of Rights focuses on the patient-doctor relationship, and the patient's responsibility to take part in her treatment and decisions relating to it.

The following is NOT part of the Patient's Bill of Rights:

Access to all patients' healthcare records to compare treatment

Rationale: Patients have the right to privacy and all of their healthcare information must remain confidential. Patients are not allowed to view other patients' files for any reason, even if it is to compare treatment or to see a potential prognosis.

The following is NOT true of the Patient's Bill of Rights:

If you speak a language other than what the Bill of Rights is written in, you must provide your own interpreter

Rationale: Healthcare providers must be able to provide an interpreter for all patients who do not speak English. This is a right all patients have, regardless of what language they speak.

The patient does not have the right to make decisions about treatment under which circumstance:

During emergency situations when the patient is unable to make decisions right away

Rationale: During emergency situations, doctors will do what is best for the patient to keep him alive and stable. Rights are never taken away due to age, any diseases the patient may have, or if he signs his care over to a family member. He still has the right to make decisions about his treatment until he is no longer physically and/or mentally capable.

The following is a patient responsibility as outlined in the Patient's Bill of Rights:

To know what medications she is currently taking

Rationale: Patients have the responsibility of knowing their past medical history, as well as what kind of medications they are currently taking. They also should know about past hospitalizations, surgeries, and anything else related to their health status.

The following is NOT a patient right:

The right to receiving emergency treatment within one hour of arrival at an ER

Rationale: The right to treatment within one hour of arrival at an ER is not a right outlined in the Bill of Rights. It does state that all patients have the right to emergency medical treatment, but the time frames are not outlined in the Bill.

Making sure the patient is living a healthy lifestyle and making healthy choices is the responsibility of:

The patient

Rationale: Patients are responsible for knowing that how they live their lives affects their personal health. Physicians and nurses should also remind and educate patients on their lifestyle choices and how these choices affect their health.

Having a copy of a patient's advanced directive on file at the hospital or physician's office is the responsibility of:

The patient

Rationale: The patient is responsible for making sure the hospital and physician's office have copies of any advanced directive she may have. If the patient has a power of attorney, it is her responsibility to make sure this is on file because a patient's treatment and course of action is based on it.

The following is NOT found on the Patient's Bill of Rights:

To demand transfer to another facility if the treatment being received isn't acceptable to the patient

Rationale: Patients cannot demand that facilities transfer them because they are not getting the treatment they want. They do have the right to file a claim outlining this so it can be reviewed, but patients may not always get the treatment they want. An example of this is patients who want narcotic pain medication and physicians who don't give it to them.

The following person is responsible for being a patient advocate and mediating problems between residents and their healthcare facilities:

Ombudsman

Rationale: The ombudsman advocates on behalf of residents when it comes to their rights and wishes. He is an unbiased party who can mediate any problems or concerns about the facility or treatment that a patient may have.

----- COURSE TEST -----

1. What is the purpose of the Patient's Bill of Rights?

A. To try and reduce the amount of lawsuits between patients and their physicians

B. To establish a job outline for healthcare workers

C. To outline what part of treatment patients are and are not allowed taking part in

D. To teach patients the importance of a healthy and open patient-doctor relationship

XXXXXDXXXXX

2. Which of the following is NOT part of the Bill of Rights?

A. Access to emergency services

B. Access to all patients' healthcare records to compare treatment

C. Taking part in treatment decisions

D. Respect and non-discrimination from all healthcare providers

XXXXXBXXXXX

3. Which of the following is NOT true of the Patient's Bill of Rights?

A. If you speak a language other than what the Bill of Rights is written in, you must provide your own interpreter

B. Pain, injury, and/or illness are all legitimate reasons for an emergency room visit

C. You have the right to ask your doctor to change your record if it isn't correct

D. Patients must follow the rules and benefits of their healthcare plan

XXXXXAXXXXX

4. The patient does not have the right to make decisions about treatment under which circumstance:

A. When she is eighty years old or older

B. During emergency situations when the patient is unable to make decisions right away

C. When she has a terminal disease

D. If she signs her rights over to a family member or friend

XXXXXBXXXXX

5. The following is a patient responsibility as outlined in the Bill of Rights:

A. To only seek treatment that he can afford

B. To tell the physician only past medical history that relates to the current illness

C. To know what medications he is currently taking

D. To know what his baseline vital signs are

XXXXXCXXXXX

6. The following is NOT a patient right:

A. The right to be informed of possible charges or costs

B. Having the available resources to resolve disputes or conflicts

C. The right to receiving emergency treatment within one hour of arrival at an ER

D. The right to continuity of care between physicians

XXXXXCXXXXX

7. Making sure the patient is living a healthy lifestyle and making healthy choices is the responsibility of:

A. The patient

B. The physician

C. All healthcare providers

D. Nurse educators

XXXXXAXXXXX

8. Having a copy of a patient's advanced directive on file at the hospital or physician's office is the responsibility of:

A. The physician's office

B. The family of the patient

C. The patient

D. The medical records department

XXXXXCXXXXX

9. The following is NOT found on the Patient's Bill of Rights:

A. To demand transfer to another facility if the treatment being received isn't acceptable to the patient

B. To be transferred to another facility if the current facility is unable to provide appropriate treatment

C. The right to review tests, treatments, and diagnoses

D. To make an effort to pay all medical bills

XXXXXAXXXXX

10. The following person is responsible for being a patient advocate and mediating problems between residents and their healthcare facilities:

A. The director of nursing

B. The ombudsman

C. The state healthcare facilitator

D. The nurse

XXXXXBXXXXX

COURSE # 12 - Communication & Interpersonal Skills

It is appropriate for the nursing assistant to tell the patient's family which of the following things:

The patient ate 75% of his dinner

Rationale: You may only tell the family things that you have witnessed yourself that do not diagnose a patient. You cannot say the patient has diarrhea, for example, because this is an assessment. You must say the patient has loose stools. Only a nurse can tell the family a patient has diarrhea. You can tell the family the amount of food the patient has or hasn't eaten, their bowel and bladder habits, their mood lately, etc. Only a nurse can discuss a patient's condition with the family, and only the family can learn things about the patient with his permission.

You should communicate patient's statuses with the nurse:

As often as needed

Rationale: When there is a change in patient status, for better or worse, the nurse should be notified immediately. You should get information from the nurse at the beginning of your shift on the baseline of your patient and monitor for changes from this baseline.

The doctor calls and tells the nursing assistant to write a new order for a dressing change on Mrs. Jones' knee. You should:

Get the nurse to take the order

Rationale: Only a nurse can take a verbal order from a physician. This is a legal issue. If the physician tries to give you an order, place him or her on hold and get the nurse to take it.

Your patient sits in his room all day and appears to be depressed. You should:

Inform him about the activities going on and offer to walk him to the activity if he is interested

Rationale: Letting a patient know of activities that are going on and that his participation is wanted can make him feel more at home. Don't force him to participate in the activities, but make sure he is aware of the social activities available.

You are taking care of a patient who strikes you out of anger. You should communicate that this is inappropriate by saying:

"Please don't hit, sir. It hurts and isn't appropriate"

Rationale: Never threaten a patient or tell him you are going to medicate him if he hits again. This is illegal and is punishable in a court of law. Explain to the patient why he should not hit and that it is painful. If it continues, remove yourself from the room and tell the charge nurse what happened.

You hear a female visitor tell her husband, who is a patient, that she would like to be intimate with him. As a nursing assistant, you must:

Provide them with privacy and inform other employees that privacy is needed

Rationale: Patients have the right to be sexually active as long as it is with a consenting adult, not done in a public place, and is not revealing to others. Employees must provide privacy for them because this is a right they have.

You should inform the nurse immediately of which of the following:

Abnormal vital signs

Rationale: Abnormal vital signs should always be reported to the nurse right away. To understand what is abnormal, the nursing assistant is responsible to know what is normal, and/or what is normal for that specific patient. If the nursing assistant is unsure, the nurse should be informed so she can decide if there is a reason to be concerned.

As a nursing assistant, you will communicate with the following types of healthcare workers:

All healthcare providers

Rationale: Nursing assistants will communicate with all healthcare workers. They are usually with patients most of the time, especially during activities of daily living like bathing, eating, and toileting. They must communicate the patient's habits and moods to the rest of the staff.

When entering a patient's room, you should communicate:

Your name, title, and task you will be doing

Rationale: When entering a patient's room, always knock first and communicate your name and title and why you are entering the room. This is a common courtesy and provides him with privacy.

When giving a report to the next shift, you should give the report and communicate changes in patients by:

Walking from room to room

Rationale: Walking from room to room and physically seeing the patients is the best way to give a report to the next shift. This is important in case there is a specific change you need to show the next nursing assistant. Some facilities discourage this type of report since the discussion of patient conditions may be overheard by others.

The following people are not allowed to communicate a change in condition to a patient's family:

A nursing assistant

Rationale: Only licensed healthcare workers, such as doctors and nurses, are allowed to communicate condition changes to a patient's family. This is not only a legal issue, but a nurse or doctor will have more knowledge of the situation than a nursing assistant may have.

You see two nurses in a heated discussion in front of a patient. You should:

Ask them to take the discussion to a private area

Rationale: Whenever there is conflict between employees, this should be dealt with in a private manner outside of business hours. If it needs to be discussed immediately, it should be away from patients and their families. If you witness this occurring in front of patients and their families, ask them to go to a private place.

When communicating with a patient who is hard of hearing, you should:

Look directly at the patient

Rationale: Many hard of hearing patients can pick up on what is being said by lip movements, even if they have had no training in lip-reading. Communication while making eye contact also increases trust and respect. Always talk to a deaf patient by facing her and making eye contact. You may need to raise your voice more than normal, but do not yell at her or talk directly into her ear. Always communicate what you will be doing, even if it takes longer to explain to her than it would a patient with normal hearing.

The nursing assistant should communicate which of the following to the nurse:

The patient complaining of his roommate being verbally abusive

Rationale: Any allegations of abuse should be reported to the nurse immediately, whether they are verbal, physical, sexual, or emotional. The nurse must further investigate these claims and make any changes accordingly.

When communicating with a patient, you should not show:

Hostility

Rationale: When communicating with a patient, project only positive emotions, even if you are frustrated, angry, or sad. Whether you are upset with work or something outside of work, positive attitudes around your patient will help her feel safe and happy. If you are unable to project positive emotions, talk to your charge nurse about taking a quick break or ask to be assigned to a different patient.

When communicating with a patient, you should be:

Clear

Rationale: When speaking with a patient, always be clear and concise and do not mumble. Make eye contact. Don't cross your arms or put your hands on your hips, as this makes you appear intimidating. Use words that are appropriate for the age of the patient you are talking to. Don't use big words with children, and don't use childish words with adults.

When telling a nurse about a new wound found on one of your patients, you should include:

The patient's room number, what the wound is or looks like, and where it is located

Rationale: Due to HIPAA privacy acts, you should protect the patient's name from being revealed in case visitors or other patients can hear it. Only tell the nurse the room number, location of the wound, and what it is or what it looks like.

You are assigned to a patient who was just diagnosed with a stroke. You know this may impair your ability to communicate with the patient because:

The stroke may have interfered with his ability to talk

Rationale: When a patient has a stroke, his ability to speak may be impaired, depending on the side and area of the brain that was damaged. Speech may or may not return depending on the extent of the stroke and how quickly it was treated. Your employer should provide you with special cards for the patient to use to communicate with the staff or with a dry erase board.

You have noticed that a couple of your long-term patients often get in arguments. After reporting this to the nurse, you should:

Separate the patients

Rationale: When patients don't get along, try to keep them apart when possible. Arrange their meals at different times, take them to different activities if possible, etc. You can't force them to remain apart unless there is abuse or violence, but try to keep further arguments from happening by separating them when possible.

When talking to your patients you are NOT allowed to tell them:

Their roommates' conditions

Rationale: Due to HIPAA, you are never allowed to communicate a patient's condition, treatment, diagnosis, etc., with any other patient. This is illegal. The CNA can be fined up to $50,000 and face permanent loss of the ability to work in a healthcare environment.

----- COURSE TEST -----

1. It is appropriate for the nursing assistant to tell the patient's family members which of the following things:

A. Their mother has been diagnosed with renal disease

B. Their father ate 75% of his dinner

C. Their grandpa will need to have emergency surgery

D. Their daughter has been diagnosed with genital herpes

XXXXXBXXXXX

2. You should communicate a patient's statuses with the nurse:

A. As often as needed

B. At the end of the shift

C. Every two hours

D. Every four hours

XXXXXAXXXXX

3. The doctor calls and tells the nursing assistant to write a new order for a dressing change on Mrs. Jones' knee. You should:

A. Write the order down in the treatment book

B. Get the nurse to take the order

C. Repeat the order to the physician to verify it

D. Make him fax an order because verbal orders aren't allowed

XXXXXBXXXXX

4. Your patient sits in his room all day and appears to be depressed. You should:

A. Tell the nurse he needs an order for depression pills

B. Take the patient to the activity room and leave him there

C. Tell him what the good TV shows are and see if he will watch TV more often

D. Inform him about the activities going on and offer to walk him to the activity if he is interested

XXXXXDXXXXX

5. You are taking care of a patient who strikes you out of anger. You should communicate that this is inappropriate by saying:

A. "Don't do that again or I'll have you arrested"

B. "I'll hit you back if you do that again"

C. "Please don't hit, sir. It hurts and isn't appropriate"

D. "I will have the nurse medicate you to settle you down if you do it again"

XXXXXCXXXXX

6. You hear a female visitor tell her husband, who is a patient, that she would like to be intimate with him. As a nursing assistant, you must:

A. Tell the nurse so she can send the wife home

B. Inform the patient that this may harm him because he is sick

C. Tell them that this isn't allowed to occur in a hospital

D. Provide them with privacy and inform other employees that privacy is needed

XXXXXDXXXXX

7. You should inform the nurse immediately of which of the following?

A. Abnormal vital signs

B. A visitor seeing how the patient is doing

C. A patient complaining that the blinds need to be shut

D. A patient who's in an abnormally grumpy mood

XXXXXAXXXXX

8. As a nursing assistant, you will communicate with what type of healthcare workers?

A. Nurses and doctors

B. All healthcare providers

C. Therapy and nutritionists

D. Other nursing assistants

XXXXXBXXXXX

9. When entering a patient's room, what should you communicate to her?

A. Your name, title, and the task you will be doing

B. Your name and title

C. Your name and what you will be doing

D. Your name

XXXXXAXXXXX

10. When giving a report to the next shift, you should give the report and communicate changes in patients by:

A. Writing down information and making a copy

B. Walking from room to room

C. Giving the next shift the information in the break room

D. Documenting the information and leaving it for the next shift member to read on her own

XXXXXBXXXXX

11. Which of the following is NOT allowed to communicate changes in a patient's condition to the family?

A. A physical therapist

B. A nutritionist

C. An LPN

D. A nursing assistant

XXXXXDXXXXX

12. You see two nurses in a heated discussion in front of a patient. You should:

A. Ask them to take the discussion to a private area

B. Ask the patient if she would like to watch

C. Move the patient to a different area

D. Ask security to come break up the discussion

XXXXXAXXXXX

13. What is the appropriate way to communicate to a patient who is hard of hearing?

A. Yell at the patient

B. Speak into the patient's ear

C. Look directly at the patient

D. Just do what needs to be done because communicating will take too long

XXXXXCXXXXX

14. The nursing assistant should communicate which of the following to the nurse?

A. The patient wants the temperature in the room changed

B. The patient wants her hair to be brushed and styled

C. The patient is complaining of her roommate being verbally abusive

D. The patient wants to move to a different room because she dislikes the wallpaper

XXXXXCXXXXX

15. When communicating with a patient, which type of emotion do you NOT want to display?

A. Compassion

B. Hostility

C. Sympathy

D. Love

XXXXXBXXXXX

16. When communicating with a patient, you should:

A. Be clear

B. Be long-winded

C. Mumble

D. Avoid eye contact

XXXXXAXXXXX

17. When telling a nurse about a new wound found on one of your patients, you should include:

A. The patient's name and room number

B. The room number and location of wound

C. The patient's name, room number, and when you found the wound

D. The patient's room number, what the wound is or looks like, and where it is located

XXXXXDXXXXX

18. You are assigned to a patient who has just had a stroke. You know this may impair your ability to communicate with the patient because:

A. She is ill and won't feel like talking

B. The stroke may have taken away her ability to talk

C. She will be unconscious for three days until treatment is over

D. She will be violent and unreasonable and not want to listen to you

XXXXXBXXXXX

19. You have noticed that a couple of your long-term patients often get in arguments. After reporting this to the nurse, you should:

A. Separate the patients

B. Ask the patients to stop and check back on them later

C. Tell the patients the police will be called if they can't stop

D. Tell the patients they are acting like children and they need to grow up

XXXXXAXXXXX

20. When talking to your patients, you are NOT allowed to tell them:

A. What's for dinner

B. Whether or not they will be getting a roommate

C. Their roommates' conditions

D. The weather

XXXXXCXXXXX

COURSE # 13 - Communication and Interpersonal Skills 2

The transmission of information through verbal or non-verbal processes is called:

Communication

Rationale: Communication is a process that allows the transmission of information through verbal or non-verbal processes. To understand its function, communication can be broken down into four basic categories. The most fundamental and important form of communication is the relay of information. Our interpretation of information is happening at all times without our even realizing it. The second most important form is asking for help. Without communication, there would be no way to ask for assistance.

During verbal communication, the message is carried by:

The sound wave

Rationale: Transmission of information is done three ways, each with two parts. The first section is an information source and the transmitter. In people, the source is the person speaking, and the transmitter is the mouth. The second way is accomplished by the listener. The receiver is the ear, and the destination is the brain, which understands the message. In between the source and the receiver are the channel and the noise. The channel is the sound waves. Noise can interfere with the message. When conveying information to a patient, it is important to consider if any factors will cause confusion in understanding.

When a patient is agitated or emotional, it is best to speak:

Slowly, clearly, with a lowered voice

Rationale: To keep a sense of perspective, it is always best to assume that a patient is visiting you on one of his worst days. The patient has come because of some pressing health situation. This is going to create stress. The degree of his stress is directly proportional to his perceived or actual health problem. When a person is under a great deal of stress it affects the ability to be rational and to communicate clearly. It is always important to take an accurate history from the patient, but you may need to adapt your style depending on his mental state. If he seems agitated or emotional, speak slowly, clearly, and with a lowered voice. If a patient is upset or angry, don't let his outbursts draw a similar reaction from you. Attempt to diffuse the situation and bring the conversation back to his care.

Understanding someone else's feelings because of your own experience is known as:

Empathy

Rationale: We have all been ill, scared, or worried at one time or another. It can be easy to forget how it felt when someone else is in the same situation. But, it is exactly this understanding that can make us great at what we do. Putting yourself in another's shoes is known as empathy. Sometimes patients just need someone to listen to them. It can take time, but it is best to just let them talk. If your patient has been through a traumatic event and you are empathetic, you may receive information that no one else will get. Patients do not share all of their information equally in healthcare. An inattentive healthcare worker will not get the same history as someone who shows that she cares.

The patient can revoke an informed consent:

At any time after the document has been signed

Rationale: When a procedure involving substantial risk is presented, a number of things must be considered. Physicians generally communicate any necessary information, but other healthcare staff may explain the procedure and the information listed on the consent forms. This consent process involves several steps to make sure there is legal protection for the institution and the patient. The procedure must be described in full, including any possible risks. It must be signed before any sedation is given. The patient must be alert and of sound mind at the time of signing. If the procedure is to be performed on a minor, the parents or legal guardians must be informed and sign. Only the physician named on the consent may perform the procedure. All elements of the informed consent form must be met before the procedure is allowed to be performed. The patient's greatest power in this process is that the informed consent may be revoked at any time after the document has been signed.

Altered LOC stands for:

Altered Level of Consciousness

Rationale: Altered levels of consciousness (Altered LOC) are changes in a patient's cognitive perception and responsiveness to the environment, stimulus, and people around them. Altered LOC can be brought on by such things as head trauma, high grade fevers, and drug overdoses. The critical thing to remember is that the patient can no longer be responsible for any aspect of his own care. All explanations, commands, and questions should be clear and concise. However, just because the patient does not seem to be alert doesn't mean that he cannot understand you. It should be assumed that no matter the LOC, the patient may be able to later recall conversations that were held in his presence. Always be courteous and professional when caring for any patient who has LOC.

A method of empowering a patient to make controlled choices about his care is called:

Valid choices

Rationale: So much of a patient's stay in a hospital involves being told what is going to happen and when. There are so few opportunities for a patient to have any control over what is happening in her life at that time. For the healthcare worker, there are many opportunities to give the patient a sense of control and security. These are called valid choices. They give patients the chance to make decisions about things that they can control and have no direct impact on their care. Having a sense of autonomy helps maintain self-esteem. Give the patient control over whether or not he would like a blanket; would he like the door open or closed; would he prefer apple or orange juice? None of these will affect your job, but will help the patient feel as if his decisions are respected and supported.

The critical characteristic of the healthcare worker's attitude will always be:

Professional

Rationale: Professional attitude and behavior is expected of every healthcare worker. Treating patients and coworkers with respect is fundamental. No discrimination of any kind should be tolerated. Honest and direct communication allows for excellent patient care. Always tell a patient what to expect before providing any care or before a procedure. Allow time for questions and give an answer that the patient can understand. When treated in a courteous manner, patients are more likely to trust their caregivers and to feel less anxious. Professional attitude is also demonstrated by being neat and well-groomed.

In some Asian cultures, people smile when they are:

Uncomfortable

Rationale: In healthcare, we serve the whole community. This includes caring for all ethnicities and cultures. It is important to understand and respect these cultures in order to give appropriate care. In many Asian countries, including China, Korea, and Vietnam, people smile when they are uncomfortable or nervous. Native Americans can consider touching an invasion of their personal space. Muslims may avoid eye contact during conversation as a sign of respect. Many healthcare facilities offer diversity training so that staff members can learn how to provide respectful care to all patients.

Informing the patient about different aspects of his care as they arise is called:

Patient education

Rationale: During the care process, a patient receives ongoing information from his healthcare providers. He may not understand medical jargon, and may be hesitant to ask for explanations. We must always provide patient information in all areas of treatment. Patient education relieves anxiety and builds trust. Patients like to be informed and are eager to learn. For example, when taking vital signs, ask if the patient understands why vital signs are checked every day. When administering a shot, explain what the medication is and why the physician has ordered it. Patient education is easy to include during any patient interaction.

----- COURSE TEST -----

1. What is the transmission of information through verbal or non-verbal processes called?

A. Speech

B. Body language

C. Communication

D. Language

XXXXXCXXXXX

2. What carries the message during verbal communication?

A. The mouth

B. The sound wave

C. The listener

D. The transmission

XXXXXBXXXXX

3. How should we speak if a patient is on edge or emotional?

A. Loudly and clearly

B. Loudly, clearly, with a slow voice

C. Slowly, clearly, with a lowered voice

D. Leave the patient alone and let him calm down first

XXXXXCXXXXX

4. What is the understanding of someone else's feelings because of your own experience known as?

A. Empathy

B. Sympathy

C. Compassion

D. Sensitivity

XXXXXAXXXXX

5. When can a patient revoke an informed consent?

A. Never, it is a binding contract

B. For 24 hours after consent

C. At any time after the document has been signed

D. Only in the presence of lawyers

XXXXXCXXXXX

6. What does altered LOC stand for?

A. Altered Loss of Consciousness

B. Altered Level of Care

C. Altered Loss of Commitment

D. Altered Level of Consciousness

XXXXXDXXXXX

7. What is a method of empowering a patient to make controlled choices about her care called?

A. Valid choices

B. Patient empowerment

C. Patient care

D. Valid selections

XXXXXAXXXXX

8. What critical characteristic should a healthcare worker's attitude always convey?

A. Being outgoing

B. Being overbearing

C. Being friendly

D. Being professional

XXXXXDXXXXX

9. When do members of some Asian cultures smile?

A. When they are sad

B. When they are lonely

C. When they are scared

D. When they are uncomfortable

XXXXXDXXXXX

10. What is informing the patient about different aspects of his care as they arise called?

A. Valid choices

B. Patient education

C. Patient information

D. Patient care

XXXXXBXXXXX

COURSE # 14 - Emergency Training Scenarios

CPR/AED training is required:

Every two years

Rationale: It is a requirement for all healthcare workers to be fully trained in the use of CPR and AED. This training must be conducted on a regular basis, typically every two years, to make sure that you are still competent in the most current techniques. CPR has undergone some changes in the last several years, and AED equipment is constantly becoming more efficient and user-friendly. The healthcare facility you work for tracks your certification's expiration date and makes sure that you are getting your license updated and renewed. However, it is your responsibility to maintain certification.

CPR stands for:

Cardiopulmonary Resuscitation

Rationale: CPR, otherwise known as Cardiopulmonary Resuscitation, is a lifesaving technique performed when someone is found not breathing and/or with no detectable pulse. The current method for administering CPR is with the acronym CAB, which stands for compressions, airway, and breathing. This technique has become the main course of action because of the critical need to maintain the victim's blood flow. If the victim has collapsed because of a cardiac arrest, there should be enough oxygen remaining in the system to maintain the body's processes long enough for you to get the blood flowing again. Current training in CPR teaches that after the initial full round of compressions, you begin examination of the airway and administering the rescue breathing.

When you find a conscious choking victim, you should begin an approach called the:

Five and five

Rationale: When you find a person choking, you should administer the "five and five" approach. The first "five" refers to the back blows. You should hit the patient with the heel of your hand between his shoulder blades five times. This can sometimes be enough force to expel the FBAO, or foreign body airway obstruction. If this does not work, then perform five abdominal thrusts, which are more popularly referred to as the Heimlich maneuver. You should alternate between these two approaches until the object is expelled.

The purpose of the Heimlich maneuver is to:

Expel a foreign object

Rationale: The Heimlich maneuver is probably the most well-known lifesaving technique in the world. It was developed by Henry Heimlich in 1974. It is also called "abdominal thrusts," but the action is identical. You get behind the choking victim and place your arms around his waist. Make a fist, thumb side in, placing it just underneath the center of the rib cage. With the other hand placed on top of your first, you thrust upward and into the victim's abdomen. You repeat until the foreign body airway obstruction (FBAO) has been expelled. If the victim is unconscious, the quick upward thrusts should be done while straddling across the victim's hips with the person lying on his back on the ground.

The critical first step to perform when finding an unconscious person is:

Call 911

Rationale: If you find someone who is unconscious, not responding, not breathing, and/or with no detectable pulse, the most critical action is to call 911. If there is no one around, find a phone immediately and call 911 before returning to the victim. If you begin CPR without first alerting an emergency squad, the victim's chances of survival are decreased. Once you have called 911, quickly check to see if there is an AED nearby. If so, make sure you take it with you while you return to the victim.

Once the CPR process begins, you first proceed with:

Chest compressions

Rationale: There is a very specific order for the CPR protocol. If you encounter someone who has collapsed or is unconscious, you always call 911 or ask a bystander to do it for you. You then attempt to get a response from the victim. If there is no reaction, roll the victim onto her back to begin CPR. Start with compressions. The rate of the compressions should be 100 per minute or more. After one round of compressions, check the airway for any blockage. If there is no blockage, tilt the head back and lift the chin to prepare for rescue breathing. Begin by pinching the victim's nose shut. Taking a normal breath, create a seal around the victim's mouth with your own, and breathe two one-second long breaths while watching the victim's chest rise and fall. Continue with CAB until the paramedics or help arrive.

The rate of breaths to compressions with partnered CPR is:

2:15

Rationale: If a patient has stopped breathing, the situation requires that you perform rescue breathing. This can be done with or without a partner, and with or without equipment. If you are alone, you should administer two rescue breaths for every thirty compressions. With a partner, use two breaths for every fifteen compressions. If you have a bag valve mask, or AMBU bag, available, make sure it is secured over the victim's nose and mouth. For manual rescue breathing, ensure that the victim's head is tilted back and the chin is lifted. Pinch the victim's nose shut. Take a normal breath, create a seal around the victim's mouth with your own, and breathe two one-second long breaths while watching the victim's chest rise and fall. If there is no chest movement, the airway may be blocked.

The rate of compressions during CPR is:

100 per/minute

Rationale: While performing chest compressions during CPR, it is absolutely critical to maintain the appropriate amount of pressure and timing throughout the process. On adults, depress the chest two inches with every compression. On infants, 1.5 inches is sufficient. The rate of compressions should be 100 per minute, or 25 compressions every fifteen seconds. For appropriate pressure, always use two hands on adults, just below the nipple line, with the fingers interlaced and arms straight. This keeps the compressions consistent and unwavering to maximize results. However, even though the compressions are constant, allow the chest to completely rise before depressing again.

AED stands for:

Automated External Defibrillator

Rationale: An automated external defibrillator, or AED, is a portable device that allows the defibrillation of victims experiencing arrhythmias. Arrhythmias can lead to cardiac arrest, so this process is critical in bystander rescues. By administering an electric shock to the heart, the arrhythmia can be stopped, allowing the heart to return to a normal rhythm. Modern AEDs are now built with extremely user-friendly instructions that are vocalized from built-in speakers. These instructions explain in simple detail the step-by-step process of administering this electrical therapy. The first step is attaching electrode pads to the victim's bare chest and plugging the pads in to the main unit. The AED will then analyze the patient's rhythm. If required, you will be asked to press the "shock" button. Immediately after the shock, if there is no heartbeat, continue with CPR.

While preparing for the paramedics, the CNA can assist by:

Taking and recording vital signs

Rationale: Depending on the type of medical site you are working for, a paramedic squad may be called for patient emergencies. Calling 911 is the protocol in this event. While waiting for the squad to arrive, you may be asked to assist the nurse. Take and record all vital signs. The nurse may administer oxygen and start an IV. Patient history, vital signs, and lab data should be given to the paramedics so that they can provide this information to the hospital.

----- COURSE TEST -----

1. CPR/AED training is required:

A. Every two years

B. Every three years

C. Every year

D. Only once

XXXXXAXXXXX

2. CPR stands for:

A. Cardiacpulmonary Resuscitation

B. Cardiac Pulse Recovery

C. Cardiopulmonary Resuscitation

D. Cardiopulmonary Recovery

XXXXXCXXXXX

3. When you find a choking victim, you should begin an approach called the:

A. Five and five

B. Blow and thrust

C. Heimlich maneuver

D. Back slap

XXXXXAXXXXX

4. The purpose of the Heimlich maneuver is to:

A. Restore the heartbeat

B. Encourage the victim to breathe

C. Prepare for paramedics

D. Expel a foreign object

XXXXXDXXXXX

5. The critical first step to perform when finding an unconscious person is:

A. Chest pulse

B. Call 911

C. Begin rescue breathing

D. Attempt to get a response

XXXXXBXXXXX

6. Once the CPR process begins, you first proceed with:

A. Rescue breathing

B. Clear the airway

C. Chest compressions

D. Shake the person

XXXXXCXXXXX

7. The rate of breaths to compressions with partnered CPR is:

A. 2:15

B. 2:30

C. 2:100

D. 15:2

XXXXXAXXXXX

8. The rate of compressions during CPR is:

A. 100 per/18 seconds

B. 30 per/minute

C. 100 per/30 seconds

D. 100 per/minute

XXXXXDXXXXX

9. AED stands for:

A. Arrhythmia External Defibrillator

B. Automatic External Defibrillator

C. Automated External Defibrillator

D. Arrhythmia External Device

XXXXXCXXXXX

10. While preparing for the paramedics, the CNA can assist by:

A. Taking and recording vital signs

B. Starting an IV

C. Administering oxygen

D. Getting directions to the hospital

XXXXXAXXXXX

COURSE # 15 - Equipment Monitoring

The type of catheter used for urine drainage is called a:

Foley

Rationale: A catheter is a tube that can be inserted into the body through different access points to allow drainage, access for surgical intervention, or administering fluids or gas. Catheters are generally thin and flexible; they are known as soft caths. They can be temporary or permanent, depending on their purpose. The most common catheters are Foley catheters (to drain urine from the bladder), central venous catheters (to administer drugs, fluids, or blood through a large vein near the heart), Swan-Ganz catheters (to measure heart pressure and to determine heart function), and feeding tubes.

Anti-embolism stockings are generally placed on lower limbs to prevent:

Deep vein thrombosis

Rationale: Anti-embolism stockings are a type of elastic sleeve typically placed on the lower legs and ankles to prevent blood clot formation. The stockings work by placing varying degrees of compression on the legs and maintaining a certain level of pressure. The desired purpose is to eliminate deep vein thrombosis (DTV). A DVT can produce a blood clot that can travel to the lungs (pulmonary embolism) or to the brain (brain embolism). If this blood clot continues, it can result in necrosis (tissue death). A DVT can cause sudden death from a pulmonary embolism.

Clean catch urine samples are collected:

After the genitals have been cleaned

Rationale: A clean catch urine sample requires a specific technique to obtain an uncontaminated sample for analysis. The process differs for age groups, genders, and the patients' ability to cooperate. Regardless of the sex, a thorough cleaning of the genital area with sterile wipes is required. Once the area is clean, a small amount of urine should be released into the toilet. If the patient is able to cooperate, the flow of urine is stopped. Urination is resumed once the collection cup is in place, filling the cup halfway. At no point should the inside of the cup or lid be touched. This routine ensures that no germs from the handler's fingers or the patient's genitals contaminate the sample.

Blood in the chest cavity is known as:

Hemothorax

Rationale: With chest trauma, free air (pneumothorax), blood (hemothorax) or other fluids are released into the chest cavity. With this additional pressure, the lungs are not able to inflate enough to get oxygen to the body. Chest tubes are inserted to drain and remove these from the thorax. The chest tube is placed between the ribs into the pleural space (an area between the linings of the lung). You will sometimes be asked to monitor the substance being drained and record the amounts in the patient's chart. The chest tubes are generally kept in place until diagnostic imaging shows that lung expansion is normal.

A technique to lower a patient's body temperature is called:

Therapeutic hypothermia

Rationale: There are a number of circumstances when a patient's body temperature needs to be heated or cooled because of a medical condition. Typically the patients are cooled using a technique called therapeutic hypothermia. Water blankets or body wraps are used to maintain a constant low surface or body core temperature. This technique is utilized when a patient has experienced a period of insufficient blood flow such as after a cardiac arrest. As a certified nursing assistant, you may be asked to monitor the temperatures of the patient, both surface and internal. You should also monitor the cooling device and report any malfunction to the nurse.

Ventilators are monitored regularly by:

Respiratory therapists

Rationale: If a patient is unable to breathe without assistance or maintain an adequate blood oxygen saturation level, he will be placed on a mechanical ventilator. The ventilator is a device that moves air in and out of the lungs at a rate determined by the physician. Ventilators are always monitored by respiratory therapists. As a CNA, you may be asked to chart the saturation levels, respiration rate, or monitor the patient's mouth where the breathing tube has been inserted and taped. It is common for saliva to be present around the patient's mouth. You may be required to perform suction when necessary. Ventilator systems are generally seen in intensive care units, cardiac recovery, and emergency rooms.

The fifth vital sign is:

Pain

Rationale: Vital signs have been traditionally divided into four standard components. The components are heart rate (how many beats the heart makes in one minute), respiratory rate (how many breaths the patient takes in one minute), blood pressure (the pressure of blood against the walls of blood vessels), and temperature (an indication of possible illness or infection). A fifth vital sign, pain, has recently been added as part of medical assessment. Certified nursing assistants will be required to monitor and record these vital signs because they are critical information for the physician. Vital signs, along with the patient history, provide a complete profile for the healthcare team.

NG-Tube stands for:

Nasogastric tube

Rationale: For patients who are unable to eat, feeding tubes are put in place to provide nutrition. The most common feeding tubes are NG-tube, G-Tube, or J-Tube. The letters indicate where the tube is inserted, or the end-point of the feeding tube. NG-Tube stands for nasogastric, or nostril to the stomach. G-Tube is inserted directly through the abdominal wall into the stomach. The J-Tube can be inserted either through the nose or the abdominal wall, bypassing the stomach altogether and ending in the jejunum portion of the small intestine. The "N" can also be replaced with an "O" for oral, if the tube is placed in the mouth. For example, an OG-Tube enters the mouth and ends in the stomach. CNAs will be asked to monitor the amount of intake, examine the access site, and document these in the patient's chart. Nasal and oral tubes are meant to be temporary, as they will cause ulcerations if used long-term. A J-tube or G-tube is placed if the physician feels that long-term use will be necessary.

A-Line is the abbreviated name for the:

Intra-arterial catheter

Rationale: An intra-arterial catheter is more commonly known as an A-line. This is a system put in place to allow continuous direct blood pressure readings and constant access to the arterial blood supply for analysis. This monitoring system consists of a catheter that is inserted into an artery and is connected to very thin tubing, and a transducer. It allows for constant patient readings. These sites must be assessed for redness during every shift. Because an A-line is a direct access to the artery, extra caution is necessary when moving or rotating the patient. If ancillary departments need to interact with the patient, such as radiology during portable x-rays, always offer your assistance with moving the patient or monitoring the lines.

For patients with an IABP, the bed must be kept in the:

Low Fowler's position

Rationale: IABP stands for Intra-aortic balloon pump. These are placed into a patient when there is a complication as a result of cardiogenic shock, angina, a cardiothoracic surgery, or certain coronary artery bypass surgeries. An IABP balloon is placed into the aorta of the heart, just short of the subclavian artery. It inflates and deflates in perfect synchronization with the beats of the heart to optimize oxygen delivery. After insertion, the entire process is regulated by a computer system. The system itself should never be manipulated by anyone except a nurse and physician. A CNA must be attentive around this system because of limitations on how to move or position a patient. The patient cannot be bent forward at all, and must always be rolled. The bed must be kept at a constant twenty to thirty degree angle called the Low Fowler's position. Always ask a nurse for specific direction before assisting with these patients.

----- COURSE TEST -----

1. The type of catheter used for urine drainage is called a:

A. Foley

B. Swan-Ganz

C. CVC catheter

D. Soft cath

XXXXXAXXXXX

2. Anti-embolism stockings are generally placed on lower limbs to prevent:

A. Deep vein thrombosis

B. Pulmonary thrombosis

C. Brain thrombosis

D. Blood thinning

XXXXXAXXXXX

3. Clean catch urine samples are collected:

A. When the patient is asleep

B. After the patient has eaten

C. After the genitals have been cleaned

D. Once the patient has washed her hands

XXXXXCXXXXX

4.   Blood in the chest cavity is known as:

A. Pneumothorax

B. Hemothorax

C. Hemathorax

D. Ureathorax

XXXXXBXXXXX

5. A technique to lower a patient's body temperature is called:

A. Therapeutic hyperthermia

B. Therapeutic cardiac cooling

C. Therapeutic hypocardia

D. Therapeutic hypothermia

XXXXXDXXXXX

6. Ventilators are monitored regularly by:

A. Nurses

B. Radiologic technologists

C. Respiratory therapists

D. Certified nursing assistants

XXXXXCXXXXX

7. The fifth vital sign is:

A. Pain

B. Respiratory rate

C. Heart rate

D. Temperature

XXXXXAXXXXX

8. NG-Tube stands for:

A. New gastric tube

B. Nasogastric tube

C. Nutrition gastric tube

D. Nutrigastric tube

XXXXXBXXXXX

9. A-Line is the abbreviated name for the:

A. Artery line

B. Access line

C. Intra-arterial catheter

D. Inter-arterial catheter

XXXXXCXXXXX

10. For patients with an IABP, the bed must be kept in the:

A. Low Fowler's position

B. High Fowler's position

C. Trendelenberg

D. Standard recumbent

XXXXXAXXXXX

COURSE # 16 - Infection Control Class #2

The acronym PPE stands for:

Personal Protective Equipment

Rationale: No matter what type of patients you work with, precautions need to be taken. Are they sweating? Are they bleeding? Are they incontinent? Have they vomited on themselves? Are they coughing up sputum or blood? These may seem like obvious questions, but each situation requires a different type of protection. PPEs, or personal protective equipment, are used to create a barrier between possible infectious materials and the healthcare professional. PPE includes gloves, masks, aprons, shoe covers, full-body "bunny suits," and caps. There are different grades of PPE as well, depending on the purpose. For example, standard masks are designed to keep droplets from moving into and out of the mouth. But standard masks do not protect against TB. Tuberculosis requires a special "duck bill" mask that must be individually fitted to provide full protection.

If you come in contact with infectious materials, you must always fill out:

An incident report

Rationale: Even when wearing PPE, an exposure to infectious material can occur. For example, your glove may get torn during a patient transfer to a cart. Immediately wash the area with soap and the hottest water you can stand for at least 25-30 seconds. Then contact your shift manager and fill out an incident report. Incident reports are required by the hospital to track all accidents that occur so future events can be prevented. Incident reports also list everyone involved in case further action or treatment is necessary.

The government agency CDC stands for:

The Centers for Disease Control and Prevention

Rationale: The CDC, or the Centers for Disease Control and Prevention, is a government agency housed under the U.S. federal agency known as the Department of Health and Human Services. The purpose of the CDC is to provide health and infectious disease information to the public and healthcare agencies. The CDC tracks diseases and health threats around the world to help prevent new outbreaks. The CDC also follows and reports infection rates for all healthcare agencies, publishes weekly report news on current disease threats, and provides guidelines for immunizations. In the event of a national or urgent outbreak, the CDC issues instructions for treating infected citizens and preventing further spread of a disease.

A hospital-acquired infection is also called a:

Nosocomial infection

Rationale: Healthcare organizations around the world have been concerned about the increase in hospital-acquired infections, or nosocomial infections. A nosocomial infection occurs within 48 hours of admission, three days after discharge, or thirty days after surgery. About 90% of these infections could be prevented by using proper hand washing technique. All healthcare professionals must wash their hands before and after every patient. Approximately two million patients contract a nosocomial infection every year. The Center for Disease Control (CDC) has published that nearly 100,000 patients die from those infections each year. These infections are generally transmitted by contact with unclean hands of healthcare workers, dirty uniforms or clothing, poor sterile technique, and contaminated catheters. It is the responsibility of every healthcare employee to learn and consistently use good hand washing techniques.

In the mid-1980s, the first attempt to standardize the protection of healthcare workers was called:

Universal Precautions

Rationale: In the mid-1980s, the principle of Universal Precautions was developed. This was the first attempt to standardize the protection of the healthcare professional. Gloves, masks, aprons, and other personal protective equipment were provided for patient care to protect healthcare workers from unnecessary exposure to infection and disease. In 1996, Standard Precautions were developed to help protect the worker and the patient from the risk of transmission of both recognized and unrecognized sources of infection. Standard Precautions for unrecognized sources apply to all body fluids, blood, and secretions and excretions except sweat, mucous membranes, and damaged skin. These are possible means of transmission that should be considered in every patient encounter. Recognized sources of transmission fall into three categories: contact, droplet, and airborne. Appropriate Standard Precautions are put into place after a confirmation of a pathogen or disease in the patient.

The three steps of medical asepsis are known as:

Microbial dilution

Rationale: Medical asepsis minimizes the growth and spread of pathogens. Patients entering the hospital are in a weakened state of health. To limit exposure to additional infection, three techniques are used to protect the patient. The combination of these techniques is called microbial dilution. When used together, they reduce the chance of nosocomial infection during hospitalization. The primary method is cleanliness: a clean room and bathroom, fresh linens, towels, and gown, and proper hand hygiene by all workers who enter the room or have patient contact. The second method is the use of chemical disinfectants to eliminate pathogens on surfaces or areas such as the bathroom. Each facility will provide products, including anti-bacterial wipes for this purpose. The third technique is sterilization using heat, gas, or chemicals to kill any pathogens. Medical asepsis depends on each of these components to provide patient protection and promote healing.

Cleansing your hands with hand sanitizer will not remove:

C-Diff

Rationale: A CNA interacts with patients more than any other healthcare team member. Proper hand hygiene is the most important way to protect patients, yourself, and your co-workers from possible contamination. In the hospital setting, hand sanitizers and sinks with soap are available inside or outside every suite. All healthcare workers are required to follow hand hygiene standards, which include washing before and after any patient contact. It is critical to understand the difference between soap and water, and hand sanitizer. A guideline is that soap and water is required for anything you can see, feel, or smell. Otherwise, hand sanitizer will suffice. If you choose not to use hand sanitizer, then you must use soap and water. One type of bacterial spores that are removed by using soap and water is C-Diff. Gloves are always available and may be worn for any patient contact; all hand hygiene practices are still followed. Healthcare facilities may also ban artificial nails and limit the length of fingernails as ways to provide patient safety.

A method of surgical asepsis that takes place in a germicidal solution is:

Chemical sterilization

Rationale: Surgical asepsis, called sterilization, is the complete destruction of pathogens from medical equipment before it can be used on a patient. There are five methods of sterilization. These are chemical sterilization, gas plasma technology, the autoclave, dry heat, and conventional gas sterilization. Chemical sterilization takes place in a germicidal solution. Gas plasma technology uses a low temperature hydrogen peroxide as an alternative to conventional gas because freon and ethylene oxide can be toxic. Autoclaves use steam to sterilize equipment under pressure. Dry heat sterilizes certain sharp instruments, powders, and greasy substances in specially-designed ovens. Conventional gas sterilization is used on materials and tools that are damaged by high heat, such as rubber, electrical, or plastic equipment.

The most common color of a sterile field is:

Blue

Rationale: There are many procedures that maintain a sterile field. For example, an ER or an ICU may have a STAT situation that requires immediate insertion of a CVC line in a patient. A physician will be assisted by a nurse during these procedures. A CNA may also be called upon to assist. It is important to know the boundaries of a sterile field. The most common color for sterile fields is blue. While other colors may be used, the principle of a sterile field is the same. Everything below the waist is considered unsterile so keep your hands elevated and above your waist at all times. Crossing your arms across your chest will keep hands at the proper level. Never reach over the sterile environment for any reason. If asked to pour a solution or place an instrument into the sterile field, do not touch anything. Keep the container outside the borders of the field while pouring. When in doubt, ask the nurse for directions before doing anything.

A person who carries a pathogen for transmission to another person is called a:

Carrier

Rationale: When contaminated with unwanted pathogens, the body is referred to as a reservoir of infection. The human body is perfect for the growth and spread of disease due to the body's stable temperature, moisture, and source of nutrients. After being exposed to or having an infectious disease, a person can be a reservoir of infection without knowing it. This person, called a host, displays no symptoms of the disease yet can infect others. These hosts are known as carriers. A host isn't the only reservoir of infection to be concerned about. A more common example of a reservoir of infection is a healthcare worker with a cold or an upper respiratory infection (URI). When a healthcare worker forgets to cover his mouth when sneezing or fails to practice proper hand hygiene, other people are at risk for becoming a reservoir of infection.

----- COURSE TEST -----

1. What does the acronym PPE stand for?

A. Personnel Protective Equipment

B. Personal Personnel Equipment

C. Protective Personnel Equipment

D. Personal Protective Equipment

XXXXXDXXXXX

2. What must you always fill out if you come into contact with infectious materials?

A. An incident report

B. Human resources questionnaire

C. Management report

D. Patient accountability report

XXXXXAXXXXX

3. What does the government agency CDC stand for?

A. The Centers for Disease Control

B. The Centers for Disease Control and Protection

C. The Centers for Disease Control and Prevention

D. The Collective for Disease Control and Prevention

XXXXXCXXXXX

4. What is a hospital-acquired infection also called?

A. Hospital disease

B. In-House infection

C. Healthcare diseases

D. Nosocomial infection

XXXXXDXXXXX

5. What was the first attempt to standardize the protection of healthcare workers in the 1980s called?

A. Standard precautions

B. Universal precautions

C. Universal cautions

D. Standard cautions

XXXXXBXXXXX

6. What are the three steps of medical asepsis known as?

A. Sterilization

B. Disinfection

C. Microbial dilution

D. Pathogenic management

XXXXXCXXXXX

7. What will hand sanitizer not remove from your hands?

A. Sweat

B. Saliva

C. Dirt

D. C-Diff

XXXXXDXXXXX

8. What is a method of surgical asepsis that takes place in a germicidal solution?

A. Dry heat

B. Gas sterilization

C. Autoclave

D. Chemical sterilization

XXXXXDXXXXX

9. What is the most common color of sterile fields?

A. Blue

B. Yellow

C. Red

D. White

XXXXXAXXXXX

10. What is a person who carries a pathogen that can be transmitted to another person called?

A. Carrier

B. Fomite

C. Reservoir of infection

D. Target

XXXXXAXXXXX

COURSE # 17 - Isolation Precautions

A protective procedure that limits the spread of infection among hospitalized patients, medical professionals, and visitors is called:

Isolation

Rationale: Every medical facility has isolation protocols to prevent the spread of disease and infection among patients, medical professionals, and visitors. Pathogens can unknowingly be spread by direct and indirect contact with an infected source. Hospitals and nursing care facilities provide care for a wide range of illnesses and conditions. When caring for many patients during a shift, all staff members are responsible for minimizing risk of exposure to infection to others.

The purpose of placing an isolation sign on the door of a patient's room is to:

Alert everyone to the need for protective precautions before entering the room, and to protect the patient from the risk of exposure to additional pathogens.

Rationale: Patients may be placed on isolation precautions for a variety of illnesses as organisms can be spread through direct and indirect contact with a patient. Some patients also need protection from additional pathogens or other factors which could interfere with their treatment. This is called "reverse isolation." It is always important to use standard precautions with all patients, but there are situations when isolation is necessary to prevent the spread of infection. When isolation is ordered, a sign should be placed on the patient's door to alert anyone entering the room that isolation protocols are in place. CNAs should be aware of isolation protocols for their facilities.

The types of isolation and precaution protocols can be found in:

The Infection Control Manual

Rationale: An Infection Control Manual must be located at every facility that contains infected materials and treats infected patients. The manual should list every type of isolation, and the CNA's responsibility when caring for patients in isolation. Everyone working at a patient care facility is responsible for knowing isolation protocols and following all precautions to protect themselves and others.

You are caring for a patient who is on respiratory isolation and you enter the patient's room to assist him to the bathroom. Along with the standard precautions used with all patients, you should wear:

A mask

Rationale: Patients on respiratory isolation transmit disease through air-droplets. A few examples of infections requiring respiratory isolation are measles, chicken pox, and influenza. A mask that covers your mouth and nose should be worn during contact with a patient on respiratory isolation. The purpose is to prevent exposure to airborne organisms circulating in the air. A gown, eye-shields, and foot covers are not necessary with respiratory isolation protocols.

The most effective way to prevent the spread of infection is:

Hand washing

Rationale: Hand washing is the most effective way to prevent the transfer of infection from one person to another. Wearing gloves is important when coming in contact with secretions or body fluids, but it is never a substitute for proper hand washing before and after each patient contact.

You are caring for a patient who is on respiratory isolation and she requires an x-ray. You should:

Put a mask on the patient before transport to radiology

Rationale: Placing a mask on the patient will prevent her from transmitting airborne organisms to others. The mask acts as a protective barrier between the patient and anyone she may have contact with. A mask provides appropriate protection, and allows the patient to go to another department for treatment.

The CDC policy that mandates that healthcare workers wear gloves, gowns, masks, and protective eyewear when exposure to blood or body fluids is likely, and considers all patients potentially infectious, is called:

Universal Precautions

Rationale: Universal Precautions were first developed by the CDC in 1987 to protect healthcare workers against HIV, Hepatitis B, and other blood-borne infections. All healthcare workers currently continue to follow this standard. Treating all patients as potentially infectious no matter what the disease may be will prevent you, your patients, and your co-workers from becoming contaminated.

When leaving the room of a patient who is on isolation precautions, you should remove this first:

Gloves

Rationale: Gloves should always be removed first when leaving the patient's room. Gloves worn in an isolation room are considered to be contaminated and should not come in contact with anything, including the door handle, your eyes, or clothing. Dispose of the gloves in the designated hazardous waste receptacle inside the room. Always wash your hands before you leave the room.

After caring for a patient on isolation precautions, you should place the patient's linens:

In a plastic bag labeled hazardous

Rationale: All linens from a patient in isolation should be bagged in a hazardous materials bag inside the patient's room and transported to the laundry per policy of the facility. It is important to label the material as hazardous so any staff coming in contact with the linens will follow isolation protocol to prevent contamination or transmission of pathogens.

You are required to wear a mask when caring for a patient who is on respiratory isolation. You should get a new mask:

Each time you enter the patient's room

Rationale: The mask you wear when caring for a patient on respiratory isolation should only be worn once and then disposed of before leaving the patient's room. The mask should be changed if it becomes damp from breathing. The mask should never be lowered around your neck and then returned to your mouth and nose. The purpose of the mask is to protect you and the patient from transmitting organisms. Never wear a mask outside of the patient's room to avoid contamination of clean areas.

----- COURSE TEST -----

1. What is a protective procedure that limits the spread of infection among hospitalized patients, medical professionals, and visitors called?

A. Immunity

B. Vectors

C. Incubation period

D. Isolation

XXXXXDXXXXX

2. What is the purpose of placing an isolation sign on a patient's door?

A. To let other patients know what is wrong with him

B. Alert everyone to the need for protective precautions before entering the room, and to protect the patient from risk of exposure to additional pathogens

C. To remind the medical staff to wash their hands

D. To let the dietary staff know the patient is not allowed to eat

XXXXXBXXXXX

3. Where can the types of isolation and precaution protocols for the facility in which you work be found?

A. On the staff bulletin board

B. On the patient's chart

C. By asking the nurse

D. In the Infection Control Manual

XXXXXDXXXXX

4. If you are caring for a patient who is on respiratory isolation and you enter the patient's room to assist him to the bathroom, along with the standard precautions that you maintain with all patients, what should you wear?

A. A gown

B. A mask

C. Eye shield

D. Protective shoe covers

XXXXXBXXXXX

5. What is the most effective way to prevent the spread of infection?

A. Wearing gloves

B. Isolating patients

C. Hand washing

D. Wearing gowns

XXXXXCXXXXX

6. If you are caring for a patient who is on respiratory isolation and she requires an x-ray, what should you do?

A. Put a mask on the patient before transport to radiology

B. Have radiology come to the patient's room

C. Tell the nurse the patient can't go to radiology because she is on respiratory precautions

D. Place all other patients back in their rooms before transporting the isolated patient in the hallway

XXXXXAXXXXX

7. What is the name of the CDC policy that mandates healthcare workers wear gloves, gowns, masks, and protective eyewear when exposure to blood or body fluids is likely, and considers all patients potentially infected?

A. Sterile field

B. Universal Precautions

C. Hand washing

D. Inflammation

XXXXXBXXXXX

8. When leaving the room of a patient who is on isolation precautions, what should be removed first?

A. Gown

B. Goggles

C. Gloves

D. Mask

XXXXXCXXXXX

9. Where should you place the linens of a patient who is on isolation precautions?

A. In the trash

B. In a plastic bag labeled as hazardous

C. In the dirty linen hamper

D. In the outside dumpster

XXXXXBXXXXX

10. How often should you get a new mask when caring for a patient who is on respiratory isolation?

A. At the beginning of your shift

B. Three times per shift

C. Every five minutes

D. Each time you enter the patient's room

XXXXXDXXXXX

COURSE # 18 - Legal & Ethical Issues

You are taking care of a patient who develops new bruises after each of her son's visits. When you ask the patient about it, she denies abuse. Your next step is:

Tell the nurse your observations

Rationale: Even if a patient denies abuse, always tell the nurse so she can investigate it. It is a nursing assistant's legal obligation to inform a nurse about possible abuse. Even if uncertain, you must report your observation so it can be investigated.

Your patient isn't cooperating while you are dressing him. The following statement is appropriate:

"I would really appreciate it if you could help me put your shirt on, Mr. Jones."

Rationale: Patients should never be threatened or verbally abused, even if the nursing assistant is frustrated. Any suspected abuse, even if it is verbal, should be reported immediately to the nurse to follow up.

The following is an example of neglect:

Not changing a patient's brief because he has severe diarrhea

Rationale: Nursing assistants must provide all patients with equal and professional care, regardless of diagnosis or condition. CNAs cannot refuse to perform a job function because of an unpleasant factor. Neglect is punishable by law and a CNA's license can be revoked.

The following is not a type of abuse:

Encouraging a patient to eat

Rationale: The four types of abuse are physical (hitting, kicking, punching, slapping, neglect), emotional/mental (making someone feel sad, depressed, fearful), sexual (touching, using, or photographing someone without their consent), and financial (misappropriation of funds or property). If any of these types of abuse are witnessed or suspected, let the nurse know immediately.

You learn that another nursing assistant didn't feed her patient because that patient tends to spit when eating. You tell the nurse about this because you know that this is:

Neglect

Rationale: Nursing assistants cannot refuse to do their jobs when it compromises the safety and health of a patient. Report the incident immediately and offer to feed the patient.

Which of the following is an example of verbal abuse?

"Do not do that or I will take you to your room."

Rationale: Never threaten a patient—this is always considered verbal abuse. If you become frustrated with a patient, simply step away for a few minutes if it is safe to do so.

The following is NOT a sign of abuse:

Frequent time spent with family

Rationale: There are many signs of abuse, including physical injuries, new onset depression, fearfulness, unusual weight loss or malnutrition, broken property, and unsafe living conditions. If anything appears unusual or different, report your observation so it can be investigated.

A dementia patient states that her roommate is always hitting her. You don't see any bruises or marks on her body. You should:

Inform the nurse

Rationale: Any patient who complains of being abused has the right to have it investigated, even if she is confused or mentally ill. Even without obvious physical evidence, the patient may still be abused. The nurse will decide how to investigate these claims further.

You observe that your patient's genitals are frequently red after her family member visits. She tells you that it's normal, but you suspect something else. The first thing you do is:

Inform the nurse

Rationale: Regardless of a patient's denial, report any suspected abuse to the nurse. If you don't report it and abuse is taking place, you can be charged with neglect and lose your license to work as a nursing assistant.

You notice that your patient appears to be sucking her thumb and rocking back and forth. This is a new behavior for her. You know that a possible cause is:

Emotional abuse

Rationale: When a patient is emotionally abused, she is being threatened, belittled, or controlled by a caregiver or family member. This can cause her to seek relief from anxiety by reverting back to childhood comforts such as thumb-sucking. Report these findings to the nurse immediately.

----- COURSE TEST -----

1. You are taking care of a patient who develops new bruises after each of her son's visits. When you ask the patient about it, she denies abuse. What is your next step?

A. Leave the subject alone since she denied abuse

B. Confront the patient's son

C. Ask the patient again later

D. Tell the nurse your observations

XXXXXDXXXXX

2. Your patient isn't cooperating while you are dressing him. The following statement is appropriate:

A. "I would really appreciate it if you could help me put your shirt on, Mr. Jones."

B. "Please help me put your shirt on or you will not go to any activities today."

C. "If you don't help me put your shirt on, the nurses are going to think you're stupid."

D. "Put your shirt on now or you'll be topless the rest of the day."

XXXXXAXXXXX

3. Which of the following is an example of neglect?

A. Not answering a call light for five minutes because you were busy with another patient

B. Not changing a patient's brief because he has severe diarrhea

C. Getting a patient up early to get him ready for a doctor's appointment

D. Taking your patient to the dining room five minutes late because you were with another patient

XXXXXBXXXXX

4. Which of the following is not a type of abuse?

A. Physical

B. Sexual

C. Encouraging eating

D. Emotional

XXXXXCXXXXX

5. You find out that another nursing assistant didn't feed her patient because that patient tends to spit when eating. You tell the nurse about this because you know that this is:

A. Mental abuse

B. Neglect

C. The nutritionist's job

D. Physical abuse

XXXXXBXXXXX

6. Which of the following is an example of verbal abuse?

A. "I need to roll you over so I can change your brief."

B. "Please do not stand up without a nurse or nursing assistant present because we don't want you to fall."

C. "If you try to walk too soon, you may need to stay in the hospital longer."

D. "Do not do that or I will take you to your room."

XXXXXDXXXXX

7. Which of the following is NOT a sign of abuse?

A. Frequent time spent with family

B. Torn clothing

C. Over or under medicating

D. Significant withdrawals from a patient's bank account

XXXXXAXXXXX

8. A dementia patient states that her roommate is always hitting her. You don't see any bruises or marks on her body. You should:

A. Know that patients with dementia often make things up

B. Ask the roommate about the allegation

C. Inform the nurse

D. Tell the patient she is only imagining things

XXXXXCXXXXX

9. You observe that your patient's genitals are frequently red after her family member visits. She tells you that it's normal, but you suspect something else. What should you do first?

A. Ask the family member to come in for a meeting

B. Inform the nurse

C. Examine the patient

D. Call the police

XXXXXBXXXXX

10. You notice that your patient appears to be sucking her thumb and rocking back and forth. This is a new behavior for her. This could be a sign of:

A. Physical abuse

B. Dementia

C. Emotional abuse

D. Neglect

XXXXXCXXXXX

COURSE # 19 - Medical Terminology

You have been assigned to care for a 75-year-old female. The physician has ordered blood glucose testing to be done ac and hs. You understand that "ac and hs" means:

Before meals and at bedtime

Rationale: Both terms are Latin, as "ac" means before meals and "hs" means hour of sleep, or bedtime.

Your patient sees an "NPO" sign over his bed and asks you what it means. The correct response would be:

Nothing by mouth

Rationale: NPO comes from the Latin phrase "nil per os" which means nothing by mouth.

The abbreviation that means "stroke" is:

CVA

Rationale: The abbreviation "CVA" stands for cerebral vascular accident. It is the medical term for a stroke. A stroke is also called a "brain attack." A CVA refers to brain damage caused by a sudden disruption of the blood supply to an area of the brain. Without blood and oxygen, brain cells quickly die. Where the stroke occurs determines the extent of damage and the prognosis for recovery. The two major types of stroke are ischemic (caused by a blood clot) and hemorrhagic (caused by a ruptured artery).

A term used in healthcare that refers to daily self-care activities is:

ADL

Rationale: Activities of Daily Living, or ADLs, are the tasks we do to take care of ourselves without assistance. Being able to perform ADLs allows people to live independently for as long as possible. Important areas of ADL are dressing, bathing, eating, continence, toileting, and transferring. Patients may be evaluated in their ability to perform these everyday tasks. A plan of care is developed for each patient to both encourage participation and to maintain safety.

"I & O" means:

Intake and Output

Rationale: Measuring intake and output is an important CNA responsibility. The process involves accurate recording of all the fluid that goes into the patient and the fluid that leaves the body. Intake includes drinks (water, milk, juice, coffee, ice chips), IV fluids, or NG/PEG tube feedings. Output includes urine, diarrhea, vomit, and occasionally blood or drainage from wounds. An accurate I & O is important for monitoring hydration and electrolyte balance, as well as some medical conditions, such as heart failure.

When giving cardiopulmonary resuscitation, the three steps are CAB, which stands for:

Compressions, Airway, Breathing

Rationale: When someone collapses, always call 911, or yell for someone nearby to do it. Determine if the person is responsive to touch or to your voice. Shake him and ask, "Are you okay?" If no response, roll the person on his back. Start with chest compressions. The most important step is to keep blood circulating. Place both hands on the center of the chest, with fingers interlaced. Push hard and fast—about one hundred times per minute for bystanders with no training. If you are trained in cardiopulmonary resuscitation (CPR), give 30 compressions and then open the airway by tilting the person's head back and lifting his chin. Pinch his nose closed and cover his mouth with yours. Give two breaths of one second each, watching to see if the chest rises. Continue with 30 compressions and two breaths until the paramedics arrive.

AEDs have been installed in many public locations, such as schools, malls, and airports. AEDs serve a role in expanding the number of opportunities for life-saving defibrillation. AED stands for:

Automated External Defibrillator

Rationale: AED stands for Automated External Defibrillator. It is a portable device that automatically analyzes the heart rhythm. If a life-threatening irregular rhythm is detected, the AED delivers an electrical-shock that restores the normal cardiac rhythm.

The doctor has written orders for vital signs to be assessed every four hours. Which of the following terms refers to this order?

VS q 4 hrs

Rationale: VS stands for vital signs, which includes temperature, pulse, respiration, blood pressure, and pain level. The q in medical terminology means "every," so the order is correctly interpreted "vital signs every four hours." The physician will determine how often vital signs should be taken for specific conditions or procedures.

The doctor has ordered for your patient to undergo a CT scan. CT stands for:

Computerized Tomography

Rationale: CT scans (sometimes referred to as CAT scans) are special x-rays used to obtain cross-sectional images of the body. CT scans of internal organs, bones, soft tissue, and blood vessels provide better images than regular x-ray exams. CT scans are used for diagnosing, locating, and following a disease or injury.

The following is true:

One cc (cubic centimeter) = One ml (milliliter).

Rationale: A cc and an ml are equivalent measurements related to volume. The metric system allows for easy conversion between liquids and solids. The volume of fluid that fits in one cubic centimeter equals one milliliter.

----- COURSE TEST -----

1. You have been assigned to care for a 75-year-old female. The physician has ordered blood glucose testing to be done ac and hs. You understand that "ac and hs" means:

A. With meals

B. Four times a day

C. Before meals and at bedtime

D. In the morning and after each meal

XXXXXCXXXXX

2. Your patient sees an "NPO" sign over his bed and asks you what it means. You should tell him:

A. Non-profit organization

B. Nothing by mouth

C. Neoplastic organism

D. No pressure orders

XXXXXBXXXXX

3. The abbreviation that means "stroke" is:

A. CVA

B. STK

C. ABD

D. CDA

XXXXXAXXXXX

4. A term used in healthcare that refers to daily self-care activities is:

A. HOB

B. SOB

C. TIA

D. ADL

XXXXXDXXXXX

5. "I & O" means:

A. Intelligence and Operations

B. Inside and Outside

C. Intake and Output

D. Important and Observations

XXXXXCXXXXX

6. What does CAB mean when giving cardiopulmonary resuscitation?

A. Cardiac, Artery, Blood

B. Continue, Always, Breathing

C. Compressions, Airway, Breathing

D. Call, Assist, Bandage

XXXXXCXXXXX

7. AEDs have been installed in many public locations, such as schools, malls, and airports. AEDs serve a role in expanding the number of opportunities for life-saving defibrillation. AED stands for:

A. Automatic External Discogram

B. Apparent Ectopic Diencephalogram

C. Automated External Defibrillator

D. Automatic Elevated Draft

XXXXXCXXXXX

8. The doctor has written an order for vital signs to be assessed every four hours. Which of the following terms refers to this order?

A. ROM

B. VS q 4 hrs

C. BID

D. QID

XXXXXBXXXXX

9. The doctor has ordered your patient to undergo a CT scan. CT stands for:

A. Control Testing

B. Cancer Transfer

C. Computerized Tomography

D. Compensatory Time

XXXXXCXXXXX

10. Which of the following is true?

A. One cc (cubic centimeter) = one second

B. One cc (cubic centimeter) = one ml (milliliter)

C. One cc (cubic centimeter) = ten cc (cubic centimeters)

D. Six hundred seconds = twenty minutes

XXXXXBXXXXX

COURSE # 20 - Medical Terminology 2

The acronym AAA stands for:

Abdominal Aortic Aneurysm

Rationale: An abdominal aortic aneurysm (AAA, or "Triple A") is a serious defect of the artery that delivers oxygenated blood to the abdomen, pelvis, and lower extremities. When the wall of the aorta weakens, it can cause the area to enlarge like a balloon. This weakening is usually gradual and a physician will closely monitor it. It can also be a sudden tear of the arterial wall, which causes life-threatening bleeding and requires immediate surgery. A male over 60-years-old is at greatest risk for an AAA.

The acronym AMA stands for:

Against Medical Advice

Rationale: Any patient who leaves a medical facility without a physician's discharge order is considered AMA, or "against medical advice."
There are several reasons for choosing to leave before treatment is completed: the inability to pay the hospital bill, drug or alcohol dependency, need to return to work or family, or disagreement with the care plan. Leaving AMA is not illegal, however, the patient is required to sign a document that releases the facility from liability.

The acronym ABG stands for:

Arterial Blood Gases

Rationale: If someone comes to the hospital with respiratory distress such as COPD, asthma, or suspected carbon monoxide poisoning, the physician may order an arterial blood gas (ABG) to measure the oxygen and carbon dioxide levels in the blood. An ABG is an important test that tells the physician how much oxygen therapy to give the patient. ABGs also measure the pH (acid - base) level in the blood. Some conditions, such as diabetes, drug overdose, or kidney disease can affect the pH result. The blood sample is taken from an artery by a specially trained respiratory therapist, lab technician, physician, or nurse.

The acronym BMI stands for:

Body Mass Index

Rationale: The Body Mass Index (BMI) is a way of determining the percentage of body fat in adults. By using a formula based on height and weight, a reliable muscle:fat ratio is calculated. A normal BMI is 18-24.9; overweight is 25-29.9; obese is 30 or more. The higher the BMI, the greater the risk for health problems, such as heart disease and type 2 diabetes.

The acronym BX stands for:

Biopsy

Rationale: A biopsy (BX) is a small piece of tissue or a few cells removed from the body and sent to the laboratory for examination or testing. A BX is the best way to determine if cancer is present. The diagnosis is made by a pathologist, a physician who specializes in analyzing tissue. Biopsies can be done on any part of the body. Some common biopsies include skin and mole, breast, colon, and bone.

The acronym CAD stands for:

Coronary Artery Disease

Rationale: Coronary Artery Disease (CAD) occurs when the main blood vessels that supply the heart muscles with oxygen and nutrients become damaged. CAD is caused by a gradual build-up of plaque and cholesterol, making the arteries hard and narrow. Without an adequate blood supply, a person with CAD may experience chest pain (called "angina") and shortness of breath. If any of the coronary arteries becomes completely blocked, the result is a heart attack. Some people don't know they have CAD until a heart attack occurs. CAD is the primary cause of death for both men and women.

The acronym COPD stands for:

Chronic Obstructive Pulmonary Disease

Rationale: Chronic Obstructive Pulmonary Disease, or COPD, is a lung disease that gets worse over time. With COPD, the lungs become stiff, or the tiny air sacs that exchange oxygen and carbon dioxide are destroyed. When air has difficulty moving in and out of the lungs, a person has shortness of breath and wheezing. Coughing produces large amounts of mucus. With limited oxygen, a person becomes tired and unable to be active. As the disease progresses, the physician may order supplemental oxygen; the patient wears a nose cannula and uses a portable oxygen tank in order to breathe more easily. The major cause of COPD is smoking. COPD is the third leading cause of death in the United States.

The acronym DNR stands for:

Do Not Resuscitate

Rationale: When a patient has no chance for recovery or a return to an acceptable quality of life, the patient, his family, or his Healthcare Power of Attorney can request an order for "Do Not Resuscitate," or DNR. A DNR is also called a "No Code." After discussing the decision, the physician will write the DNR order in the patient's chart. The person responsible for the decision may be asked to sign a form that is also placed in the patient's chart. A DNR order means that no CPR will be performed if the patient's heart stops beating or if he stops breathing. Making a DNR decision can be difficult. Patients and families may require emotional support during and after the decision. A DNR order can be rescinded at any time.

The acronym DX stands for:

Diagnosis

Rationale: A diagnosis (DX) is the identification of a disease or condition. Physicians determine a diagnosis by examining symptoms, as well as lab, biopsy, x-ray, and CT results. When being admitted to the hospital, a patient will have an "admitting diagnosis." This diagnosis may remain the same or it may change, depending on test results. The diagnosis will determine the plan of care during the hospital stay. At discharge, the physician will provide a "final diagnosis."

The acronym ERCP stands for:

Endothermal Retrograde Cholangio-Pancreatography

Rationale: In the event a patient has been complaining of abdominal pain that has become frequent and without relief, an ERCP, or endoscopic retrograde cholangio-pancreatography exam, may be ordered. This exam involves many different areas of the hospital working in sync to obtain a diagnosis or resolution of the patient's diagnosis. A long, flexible light with a camera attached is sent into the mouth. With the assistance of fluoroscopy (live x-ray) the endoscope is guided down the esophagus, through the stomach, and into the duodenum to a point where it connects with the pancreatic ducts. At this point, the physician can use imaging to determine many different problems with the patient. The more common are gallstones that can usually be removed during the procedure, but biopsy samples can be taken and stents can even be put in place if necessary.

The acronym PRN stands for:

Pro Re Nata

Rationale: PRN comes from a Latin phrase, "Pro Re Nata." It means "as needed" or "as necessary." Example: Physicians may write an order for "Tylenol q 4 hrs PRN." This means that the nurse can give the patient some Tylenol every four hours, if needed. The decision is left to the nurse. For a CNA, there may be orders such as: ambulate PRN, out of bed PRN, or ice chips PRN.

----- COURSE TEST -----

1. What does the acronym AAA stand for?

A. Abdominal Aortic Aneurysm

B. Abdominal Aortic Aeration

C. Arterial Abdominal Aneurysm

D. Aortic Arterial Aneurysm

XXXXXAXXXXX

2. What does the acronym AMA stand for?

A. Against Medical Advice

B. Abdominal Metastatic Aneurysm

C. Against Medical Admission

D. Aortic Metastatic Aneurysm

XXXXXAXXXXX

3. What does the acronym ABG stand for?

A. Abdominal Blood Gases

B. Aortic Blood Gases

C. Arterial Blood Gases

D. Arterial Blood Grading

XXXXXCXXXXX

4. What does the acronym BMI stand for?

A. Bowel Movement Indicator

B. Body Movement Indicator

C. Body Mass Index

D. Body Management Index

XXXXXCXXXXX

5. What does the acronym BX stand for?

A. Bacteria

B. Biopsy

C. Blood Gases

D. Benign

XXXXXBXXXXX

6. What does the acronym CAD stand for?

A. Cardiac Artery Disease

B. Coronary Artery Disease

C. Celiac Artery Disease

D. Cardiac Ascension Development

XXXXXBXXXXX

7. What does the acronym COPD stand for?

A. Chronic Obstructive Pulmonary Disease

B. Chronic Obstructive Pulmonary Defibrillation

C. Chronic Obstructive Primary Disease

D. Clear Obstruction Pulmonary Disease

XXXXXAXXXXX

8. What does the acronym DNR stand for?

A. Do Not Revive

B. Damage Negates Recovery

C. Do Not Resuscitate

D. Do Not Reveal

XXXXXCXXXXX

9. What does the acronym DX stand for?

A. Diagnosis

B. Drainage

C. Department

D. Determined

XXXXXAXXXXX

10. What does the acronym PRN stand for?

A. Pro Re Nata

B. Per Registered Nurse

C. Physician-Requested Nursing

D. Pro Resuscitation Needs

XXXXXAXXXXX

COURSE # 21 - Modern Communications

Cell phone use can be restricted in hospitals because of:

Patient privacy

Rationale: While cell phones generally do not interfere with monitoring equipment, hospitals may restrict cell phone use in patient areas for several reasons. Protection of patient privacy is a hospital responsibility; with current cell phones able to take photos and videos, there is a serious risk of HIPAA violation. A hospital may allow cell phones to be used in general areas, such as the waiting room, lobby, or cafeteria. Cell phone use can also be disruptive to ill patients who are trying to sleep or rest, and can interfere with care or treatments. A third reason is that cell phones are not allowed in intensive care units or areas that use monitors and high-tech equipment. Every hospital employee should be familiar with the policy regarding cell phone use.

For emailing to be safe in the hospital environment, it must undergo a process called:

Encryption

Rationale: Encryption is the scrambling, or "encoding" of information into a text that can only be read by authorized people. Any medical institution that uses email containing Protected Health Information (PHI) must encrypt the PHI to protect patient privacy. HIPAA, the Health Insurance Portability and Accountability Act, has enacted specific precautions and security standards that all medical institutions must follow, including encryption of PHI. Violation of any HIPAA standard can result in a severe financial penalty for a healthcare facility.

A directive given by a physician or other qualified healthcare team member that contains a specified medication, treatment, or test is called an:

Order

Rationale: Every function of a healthcare worker's job is the result of an order in a patient's chart. Physicians, nurse practitioners, and physician's assistants can all write orders into a patient's chart. These orders can be communications to any department within the healthcare facility. The orders can be requests for anything necessary to diagnose or treat the patient, such as blood work, urinalysis, diagnostic imaging, or medications. A verbal order can only be given to a nurse. The nurse will enter it into the chart, but it must be signed by the physician within 24 hours.

The summary of treatment and the instructions given to the patient before leaving the hospital are called the:

Discharge paperwork

Rationale: Discharge paperwork is one of the final steps before leaving a healthcare facility. A physician or nurse meets with the patient and family to give them a final diagnosis and summary of treatment received during hospitalization. The patient also receives clear aftercare instructions, including any medications prescribed for home use. Discharge paperwork also provides recommendations for making appointments with a PCP or a specialist, symptoms to watch for when home, and instruction to visit an ER if pain or other symptoms return or get worse. Included with the discharge package should be any prescriptions for medication or referrals for additional treatment.

A secure messaging system that allows for a physician and patient to communicate is called:

Web messaging

Rationale: Physicians cannot always be available to speak with a patient who is seeking information, advice, or reassurance. The development of web messaging allows for private and secure communication between physician and patient. These communications are encrypted over a network that allows email, video, and wireless conferencing from any web browser. This system also allows nurses and healthcare professionals to communicate easily and efficiently.

The documents required before a scheduled admission or non-emergency treatment in a healthcare facility, including medical consent, contact information, billing and insurance information, and advance directives are called:

Admission paperwork

Rationale: When a patient enters the hospital for surgery or treatment, the first stop is at the Admissions Department. A nurse or coordinator will provide information about the scheduled procedure, obtain informed consent, and collect necessary details about insurance or payment. Advance directives, such as a Living Will or Healthcare Power of Attorney, are copied and added to the patient's file. The patient receives a copy of this admission paperwork, which includes instructions regarding the stay, what to bring, and information for visitors. Patients who enter the hospital through the Emergency Department may be treated and admitted before providing any information. At a reasonable time, an ER representative will obtain the necessary information and provide the patient and/or family with admission paperwork.

The extensive electronic file of information about an individual's medical history, including treatments, imaging reports, diagnoses, medications, and lab reports is called an:

Electronic Health Record

Rationale: The medical chart is the most critical component for a patient's healthcare team. In a hospital setting, an electronic health record (EHR) is the current standard for documenting a patient's care. All treatments, medications, and progress notes are available within the healthcare setting. The EHR can also be shared with other providers, which allows a patient's comprehensive medical chart to be viewed by authorized staff. Since the EHR can be widely shared, accuracy is important. A current EHR allows for better treatment, fewer duplications, and clinical efficiency.

A chart used as a quick, graphical reference for vital signs, lab results, and I & O is called a:

Flow sheet

Rationale: A flow sheet provides a 24-hour view of significant information about a patient at regular intervals so the physician and healthcare team can quickly track the patient's condition. The flow sheet contains data such as vital signs, oxygen saturations, lab results, and intake/output. As with all charting, accuracy is critical to maintaining a state of proper patient care. All flow charts are included in the permanent medical record.

A system for cataloging patient information so that it is easily retrievable in the future is called:

Medical records

Rationale: Every medical facility will have its own system of cataloging patient information. This system is called medical records. No matter how large or small the medical facility, the same standards apply. Medical records must include patient name and demographic information, unique identification number, record of treatments, laboratory and test results, medications, and progress notes. Each facility can determine a system for obtaining medical records. Small facilities may file alphabetically. A large hospital or healthcare system may have an electronic data base.

The acronym PHI stands for:

Protected Health Information

Rationale: PHI stands for Protected Health Information. PHI stands for any of the eighteen identifiers that can be linked to an individual patient, such as name, address, date of birth, and Social Security number. It also includes any health information such as medical record numbers, and dates of admission, discharge, or death. PHI that is recorded in any form, by any health system, at any time, must be secured.

----- COURSE TEST -----

1. Cell phone use in hospitals is restricted because of:

A. Patient privacy

B. Union rules

C. Violation of the Cell Phone Act

D. Microsoft policy

XXXXXAXXXXX

2. What process must email undergo to be safe in the hospital environment?

A. Encryption

B. Decryption

C. The lock and key system

D. Stamping

XXXXXAXXXXX

3. What is a directive given by a physician or other qualified healthcare team member that contains a specified exam, medication, or treatment called?

A. Rationale

B. Objective

C. Job

D. Order

XXXXXDXXXXX

4. What is the final set of recommendations and instructions for the patient, and the last documents entered in the chart before the patient leaves the hospital called?

A. Exit instructions

B. Exit paperwork

C. Disconnection paperwork

D. Discharge paperwork

XXXXXDXXXXX

5. What is a secure messaging system that allows for physician to patient communications called?

A. E messaging

B. Web messaging

C. Internet messaging

D. Web texting

XXXXXBXXXXX

6. What are the documents required before non-emergency treatment in a healthcare facility, including medical consent, contact information, billing information, insurance information, and legal paperwork, called?

A. Entrance paperwork

B. Admission protocols

C. Admissions paperwork

D. Entrance protocols

XXXXXCXXXXX

7. The extensive electronic file of information about an individual's medical history, including treatments, imaging reports, diagnoses, medications, and lab reports, is called an:

A. Excel spreadsheet history

B. External historic record

C. Electric hard drive

D. Electronic health record

XXXXXDXXXXX

8. What is a chart that is used as a quick, graphical source to review itemized vital signs, lab results, and tests ordered called?

A. Order flow

B. Flow sheet

C. Order packet

D. Flowchart

XXXXXBXXXXX

9. A system for cataloging patient information so that it is easily retrievable in the future is called:

A. Medical records

B. Doctor's records

C. Patient records

D. Filing records

XXXXXAXXXXX

10. What does the acronym PHI stand for?

A. Public Health Information

B. Public Health Initiative

C. Protected Health Information

D. Protected Health Initiative

XXXXXCXXXXX

COURSE # 22 - Patient Condition

A heart attack is also known as a:

Myocardial Infarction

Rationale: A myocardial infarction (MI), or heart attack, is a medical emergency. It happens when blood flow to the cardiac muscles is blocked. The heart has two main coronary arteries that provide blood and oxygen to the entire heart. If the coronary arteries become obstructed by a blood clot, the portion of the heart muscle at the point of the obstruction will die. Blood clots are the result of thickening and narrowing of the arteries by plaque. Plaque is a waxy substance made from cholesterol.

A stroke is also referred to as a:

Brain attack

Rationale: A stroke or "brain attack" is a medical emergency, similar to a heart attack. A stroke occurs when the brain is suddenly deprived of blood flow. If the brain doesn't receive a constant supply of blood, the brain cells begin to die from the lack of oxygen. There are two main types of strokes: ischemic and hemorrhagic. Ischemic strokes are caused by arteries obstructed by plaque, forming a blood clot in a vessel that supplies blood to the brain. A hemorrhagic stroke takes place when a weakened blood vessel leading into the brain ruptures, leaking blood directly into the brain.

When a foreign substance is inhaled, it is called:

Pulmonary aspiration

Rationale: Pulmonary aspiration occurs when someone breathes in a foreign substance, such as food, liquid, medicine, or vomit. Aspiration can occur two ways. First, a patient may swallow incorrectly, sending the substance into the trachea instead of the esophagus. The second way is from the stomach, back up the esophagus. The danger of foreign materials entering the lungs is that aspiration pneumonia can develop. Aspiration is more common in geriatric patients. The CNA should remain with elderly patients during meal times and make sure diet orders are being followed.

The most common fracture following the fall of an elderly patient is a:

Hip fracture

Rationale: Preventing falls is a priority in every hospital and healthcare facility. Injuries from falls can have serious consequences, and require surgery, extended hospitalization, or rehabilitation. Elderly patients are more likely to break their hips in a fall, depending on age and health status, and a fall can result in death.

A lung infection is known as:

Pneumonia

Rationale: Pneumonia is an infection in one or both lungs. It is caused by bacteria, viruses, or fungi. Patients at risk for developing pneumonia include those with compromised immune systems or chronic lung diseases, recent surgery, and smokers or alcoholics. Two ways of contracting pneumonia are community-acquired pneumonia and nosocomial infection. Community-acquired pneumonia develops from exposure in social settings or public places, such as school, work, or shopping malls. Nosocomial infections are acquired from a hospital or healthcare institution. Proper hand washing is the primary prevention method.

A fracture that breaks through the skin is called an:

Open fracture

Rationale: A fracture is a broken bone. There are two types of fractures, open and closed. In an open fracture, the broken bone punctures the skin, causing a wound. Open fractures require immediate attention. Surgery will be necessary, along with antibiotics to prevent infection. Open fractures are usually the result of trauma, such as motor vehicle accidents, sports injuries, or falls. Closed fractures do not puncture the skin.

A degenerative change in the brain that causes impairment is called:

Dementia

Rationale: Dementia is a chronic brain disorder that interferes with the ability to perform routine or daily tasks. The degenerative changes lead to impairment of language, memory, emotions, perception, and cognition. Dementia can be the result of traumatic brain injury or stroke, or diseases such as Alzheimer's and Multiple Sclerosis. The first symptoms generally displayed are forgetfulness or difficulty accomplishing simple tasks. Dementia can progress into getting lost in familiar areas, speech difficulty, and personality changes. The condition can become so extreme that the patient will no longer be able to recognize her own family, feed herself, or use the bathroom without assistance. A great deal of patience and understanding is required when working with a patient suffering from dementia.

The fourth level of consciousness is:

Comatose

Rationale: During the assessment of a patient, there is an opportunity to measure her awareness of the immediate environment. To properly categorize this, the four levels of consciousness were developed. This is a quick way to communicate if a patient seems to be stable, or if she requires immediate medical attention. The first LOC is alert and conscious. Patients are aware of their surroundings and can answer questions without distraction. The second LOC is drowsy but responsive. The patient may be extremely lethargic, but will eventually answer questions if given some time. The third LOC is unconscious but responsive to painful stimulation. The patient is incapable of answering any questions, but the body will react to pain. The fourth LOC is comatose. The patient is completely incapacitated and does not respond to questioning or stimulus of any kind.

The maneuver used to help a choking victim is called the:

Heimlich maneuver

Rationale: Choking is an obstruction of air flow into and out of the lungs. This blockage can be total or partial, and can be caused due to a foreign body (such as food) or from swelling in the throat (laryngeal edema). If you happen upon a conscious patient choking, always look in the mouth first to visualize the blockage. The Heimlich maneuver should be performed immediately.

The term used to describe light-headedness is:

Orthostatic hypotension

Rationale: Orthostatic hypotension is the sudden drop in blood pressure that results from suddenly standing up. It usually resolves within a few seconds to a minute. If it happens frequently, a physician should be consulted. Some causes for frequent orthostatic hypotension are dehydration, diabetes, heart disease, getting up too quickly after eating, and some nervous system disorders.

----- COURSE TEST -----

1. A heart attack is also known as a:

A. Heart infarction

B. Myocardial infarction

C. Myocardial infraction

D. Aortic trauma

XXXXXBXXXXX

2. A stroke is also referred to as:

A. An aneurysm

B. An occipital meltdown

C. A brain attack

D. Ischemia

XXXXXCXXXXX

3. When a foreign substance is inhaled, it is called:

A. Pulmonary aspiration

B. Coronary aspiration

C. Aspiration

D. Aortic aspiration

XXXXXAXXXXX

4. The most common fracture following the fall of an elderly patient is a:

A. Nose fracture

B. Knee fracture

C. Leg fracture

D. Hip fracture

XXXXXDXXXXX

5. A lung infection is known as:

A. Pneumonia

B. Nosocomial infection

C. Community acquired infection

D. Strep

XXXXXAXXXXX

6. A fracture that breaks through the skin is called:

A. A non-displaced fracture

B. An open fracture

C. A displaced fracture

D. A closed fracture

XXXXXBXXXXX

7. A degenerative change in the brain that causes impairment is called:

A. Stroke

B. Myocardial infarction

C. Dementia

D. Brain attack

XXXXXCXXXXX

8. The fourth level of consciousness is:

A. Alert and conscious

B. Drowsy but responsive

C. Comatose

D. Unconscious but responsive to pain

XXXXXCXXXXX

9. The maneuver used to help a choking victim is called the:

A. Heimlich maneuver

B. Himlik maneuver

C. Hemill maneuver

D. Finger sweep

XXXXXAXXXXX

10. The term used to describe light-headedness is:

A. Orthostatic hypotension

B. Syncope

C. Orthostatic hypertension

D. Dementia

XXXXXAXXXXX

COURSE # 23 - Patient Rights

Patients have the right to:

Considerate and respectful care from all care providers

Rationale: The individual rights of patients are an important ethical principle in health care. Every patient is entitled to be treated with dignity regarding culture and beliefs.

The word "accountability" means:

Personal responsibility for one's own actions

Rationale: Accountability means to be responsible or answerable for what you do. It involves taking responsibility for your own actions and being able to explain them.

Encouraging a patient to be involved in planning and carrying out her own care supports the patient's right to:

Autonomy

Rationale: Autonomy means being free to choose. Possible patient choices include identifying goals and care measures compatible with one's culture, religion, and personal values. Considered one of the most important and fundamental of all is the patient's right to direct the medical treatment they choose to receive or reject. Patient "autonomy" or self-determination is at the core of all medical decision making in the United States.

A way to show respect for a patient's right to privacy is to:

Knock before entering the room, and announcing your presence

Rationale: Every patient has the right to privacy. Knocking on the door and letting the patient know you are coming in is respectful. A patient also has the right to restrict or refuse visitors. Besides physical privacy, a patient has the right to request a staff member of the same gender be present for an examination.

When documenting about a patient, you should:

Record all care and instructions given

Rationale: Record all interventions and instructions given to the patient. Only documented care is acceptable in a court of law. Documentation should be objective. All patient-related communication should be documented by the person who spoke with the patient. Flow sheets must be marked with detailed, exact information, along with dates and times.

A patient tells you, "I want you to bring my medical record so I can read it. I know HIPAA gives me the right to see it." You should:

Explain that you will inform your supervisor, who will follow facility policy

Rationale: The patient's request must be honored, but agency protocol must be followed in doing so. Usually a physician or RN reviews the record with the patient to translate medical terminology and answer questions. Nursing assistants should not give the patient his chart unless approved by a direct supervisor.

The term used to describe a competent patient's agreement to have a surgical procedure after the physician explains the procedure, the desired outcome, possible complications, and possible alternative treatment is:

Informed consent

Rationale: Informed consent must be obtained for invasive procedures ordered for therapeutic or diagnostic purposes. Parents cannot give informed consent for the treatment of their children, but they can authorize their treatment up to a certain age (authorized consent). Informed consent means that the patient is informed in non-medical language, or in a way that the patient can understand. If the patient does not speak English, an interpreter must be provided. The patient must also be informed that he or she has the right to revoke written permission at any time.

The nurse discusses the patient's condition on the phone with the patient's brother. Learning this, the patient is upset, saying he has not spoken with his brother for years and did not want his brother to know anything about his condition. The nurse has:

Breached confidentiality

Rationale: All medical information is strictly confidential. If the person receiving treatment is a minor, the responsible parent or guardian can determine what information to share with others. If the patient is not a minor, only the patient can decide who may receive information regarding his condition. Medical personnel may not give out information to any person regarding any patient without written consent from the patient. The patient must specifically name who may receive the information or updates.

Regarding informed consent, it is true that:

A patient has the right to revoke consent at any time

Rationale: Informed consent means that the procedure is explained to the patient in non-medical language. No matter at what stage of treatment the consent is revoked, treatment must be stopped.

While helping a patient to get out of bed and get ready for therapy, he tells you that he did not sleep well last night and just wants to go back to sleep. You remind him of the importance of attending therapy sessions, but he simply refuses to go. The first appropriate action is to:

Notify the nurse of the patient's refusal of therapy

Rationale: Patients have the right to refuse service, proposed tests, or treatment. By notifying the nurse, she can explain the anticipated medical consequences if the patient still refuses care. The patient may be expected to sign a statement refusing care. It is the nurse's responsibility to contact the physician.

----- COURSE TEST -----

1. Patients have the right to:

A. Considerate and respectful care from all care providers

B. Information about diagnosis and prognosis from the practical nurse

C. Medical care of their choice regardless of ability to pay

D. Any food requested and in as large a quantity as desired

XXXXXAXXXXX

2. What does the word accountability mean?

A. A transfer of responsibility for wrong actions

B. Shared responsibility with the physician for wrongdoing

C. Personal responsibility for one's own actions

D. Giving up responsibility when the situation allows

XXXXXCXXXXX

3. Encouraging a patient to be involved in planning and carrying out his own care supports the patient's right to:

A. Confidentiality

B. Privacy

C. Autonomy

D. Justice

XXXXXCXXXXX

4. A way to show respect for a patient's right to privacy is to:

A. Keep all items within the person's reach

B. Color code all important paperwork

C. Announce when you enter and leave the room

D. Place all furniture up against the walls

XXXXXCXXXXX

5. When documenting patient behavior, you should:

A. Record subjective interpretations of patient behavior

B. Avoid mentioning communicating with supervisors to seek advice

C. Record all care and patient instruction given

D. Summarize care in the progress notes and flow sheets

XXXXXCXXXXX

6. A patient tells you, "I want you to bring my medical record so I can read it. I know HIPAA gives me the right to see it." You should:

A. Bring the record to the patient immediately

B. Explain that you will inform your supervisor, who will follow facility policy

C. Try to talk the patient out of seeing the record by offering to answer questions

D. Tell the patient to make the request in writing to the physician

XXXXXBXXXXX

7. The term used to describe a competent patient's agreement to have a surgical procedure after the physician explains the procedure and its alternatives is:

A. Statute

B. Competency

C. Informed consent

D. Standard of care

XXXXXCXXXXX

8. The nurse discusses the patient's condition on the phone with the patient's brother. On learning this, the patient is upset, saying he has not spoken with his brother for years and did not want his brother to know anything about his condition. The nurse has:

A. Slandered the patient

B. Committed a felony

C. Breached confidentiality

D. Assaulted the patient

XXXXXCXXXXX

9. Which of the following is true regarding informed consent?

A. Informed consent must be obtained for surgical procedures only

B. Parents can give informed consent for the treatment of their children

C. Informed consent means the patient is informed in medical language

D. A patient is informed that he or she has the right to revoke consent at any time

XXXXXDXXXXX

10. If a patient refuses to attend therapy that you are preparing him for, first:

A. Call the doctor to report that the patient did not sleep well

B. Notify the nurse of the patient's refusal of therapy

C. Ignore the patient's requests and take him to therapy anyway

D. Arrange for the therapist to conduct the session in the patient's room

XXXXXBXXXXX

COURSE # 24 - Pressure Sores and Skin Tears

When skin becomes red or begins to break down due to constant rubbing or pressure, it is called a:

Pressure ulcer

Rationale: Pressure ulcers develop from reduced blood flow to an area of skin, typically by unrelieved pressure or rubbing at the site. Pressure ulcers are also called decubitus ulcers, pressure sores, or bedsores. Factors that affect skin integrity include immobility, health history, and nutrition. As a CNA, it is vital to look at the skin when performing daily tasks with patients and always notify the nurse of any redness or open areas.

The first symptom of a pressure ulcer is:

Reddened skin

Rationale: When skin remains in the same position for more than two hours, it may appear reddened. In patients with dark skin, the area may appear discolored. The patient may complain of pain or tenderness, and the area may feel warm or cool to the touch. Immediately report any red or discolored skin to the nurse.

A new pressure ulcer should first be treated by:

Relieving pressure on the skin

Rationale: The first step after identifying and reporting a reddened area is to reposition the patient to relieve pressure. As a CNA, your actions will depend on the site. You may use pillows or blankets to prop a patient on her other side, elevate her heels off the bed, or pad a railing on the bed or wheelchair. Always notify the nurse of any reddened or discolored areas, as further intervention may be needed to treat the skin.

To prevent skin breakdown, a patient should be repositioned:

Every two hours

Rationale: A patient should change position at least every two hours to prevent skin breakdown. This is most critical for patients who are immobile or unable to reposition themselves in bed. Most nursing facilities typically have a protocol and schedule to help the CNA consistently reposition patients.

Patients are more susceptible to pressure ulcers if they are:

Confined to a bed or a wheelchair

Rationale: Patients who are immobile or unable to reposition themselves are at risk for skin breakdown. It is essential to observe the skin when providing daily care to patients and to notify the nurse of any skin changes. Skin areas most prone to breakdown are the heels, buttocks, back of the head, and elbows.

A skin wound that separates the layers of skin is a:

Skin tear

Rationale: A skin tear is most common in elderly patients, as their skin is thin and fragile. These skin injuries can occur during routine care. It is important to handle the skin carefully when providing care to all patients, but especially the elderly.

Patients who are at the highest risk of a skin tear are:

Elderly patients

Rationale: Elderly patients are more prone to skin tears because skin gets thinner with age. Skin tears are traumatic injuries that occur with minimal friction to the skin. Elderly and very ill patients require special attention to prevent skin tears.

The most common cause of skin tears in the elderly occurs during:

Routine daily activities

Rationale: Skin tears in the elderly are most likely to occur during routine care such as bathing, dressing, repositioning, or transfer. Patients over eighty years old have thin, fragile skin and are at risk for injury. Preventive measures include dressing elderly patients in clothing with long sleeves and long pants. The CNA should use extra caution in all aspects of patient care, including removing tape or bandages. Always notify the nurse of any skin changes or damage.

A patient who sits for a prolonged period of time in a wheelchair is prone to skin breakdown on the:

Outer thighs and buttocks

Rationale: When a patient sits for a long period of time without a position change, pressure is put on the outer thighs and the buttocks. A patient should not be left sitting in a wheelchair for longer than two hours without being helped to stand up, walk, or repositioned. Wheelchairs should be properly sized and fitted for each patient.

In order to repel moisture and to provide a protective barrier for the skin, you may apply:

Protective cream

Rationale: A protective cream may be applied to the skin to provide a barrier against moisture and bacteria. The creams are typically applied to the peri-area to protect the skin of patients who are incontinent. Prolonged moisture weakens the skin and increases the chances of developing a pressure ulcer. The cream should only be applied at the direction of a nurse, as a nursing order may be required.

----- COURSE TEST -----

1. When skin becomes red or begins to break down due to constant rubbing or pressure, it is called:

A. Necrosis

B. A pressure ulcer

C. A blister

D. Acne

XXXXXBXXXXX

2. What is the first symptom of a pressure ulcer?

A. Reddened skin

B. Black area

C. Open sore

D. Amputation

XXXXXAXXXXX

3. What is the first thing that should be done to a new pressure ulcer?

A. Place a bandage on the area

B. Call the doctor

C. Relieve pressure on the skin

D. Have the patient get out of bed

XXXXXCXXXXX

4. How often should a patient be repositioned to prevent skin breakdown?

A. Once per shift

B. Every two hours

C. Once per day

D. At bedtime

XXXXXBXXXXX

5. What type of patients are the most susceptible to pressure ulcers?

A. Those confined to a bed or a wheelchair

B. Ambulatory patients

C. Young children

D. Pregnant females

XXXXXAXXXXX

6. What is a skin wound that separates the layers of skin?

A. A pressure ulcer

B. A scab

C. A skin tear

D. An incision

XXXXXCXXXXX

7. Which patients are at the highest risk of a skin tear?

A. Teenagers

B. Young adults

C. Diabetics

D. Elderly patients

XXXXXDXXXXX

8. When do most skin tears occur with the elderly?

A. Surgery

B. Tape removal

C. Falls

D. Routine daily activities

XXXXXDXXXXX

9. When a patient sits for a prolonged period of time in a wheelchair, she is most susceptible to skin breakdown at what site?

A. Back of the head

B. Outer thighs and buttocks

C. Elbows

D. Heels

XXXXXBXXXXX

10. What may be applied to the skin to repel moisture and to provide a protective barrier for the skin?

A. Protective cream

B. Blankets

C. Bandages

D. Water

XXXXXAXXXXX

COURSE # 25 - Pulse Oximetry & Oxygen Administration

A non-invasive procedure that measures the oxygen saturation of arterial blood is called:

Pulse oximetry

Rationale: Pulse oximetry (pulse ox) is a non-invasive procedure that measures the level of oxygen saturation in arterial blood. It is typically ordered on patients who require oxygen, or those who are at risk for low oxygen levels. A pulse ox level is obtained by placing a probe on the patient's finger. The result is displayed on the pulse ox machine. A normal oxygen saturation level is over 95. Some patients may have a lower level because of chronic illnesses, such as emphysema or COPD.

A plastic device that administers oxygen through two prongs inserted into the nostrils is called a:

Nasal cannula

Rationale: A nasal cannula is a soft, plastic device for oxygen administration, with two prongs that are inserted into the nostrils. This is the most common way that oxygen is administered to patients. The cannula does not interfere with the patient's ability to eat or speak, and can be humidified for patients who complain of dryness from wearing oxygen.

An artificial opening into the trachea is called a:

Tracheostomy

Rationale: The trachea is located in the front of the throat, and is the airway through which we breathe. A tracheostomy is an artificial airway placed directly into the trachea to allow oxygen to be administered directly into the lungs. An incision is made into the trachea, and a tube is inserted to keep the airway open. A patient with a tracheostomy may be on a ventilator. A CNA should be trained before providing trachea care.

You are caring for a patient who is on oxygen, administered through a nasal cannula at 2L per minute. When transporting the patient to the cafeteria for dinner, you should:

Place the patient on a portable O_2 tank at 2L

Rationale: When caring for a patient on continuous oxygen therapy, it is important to maintain the oxygen level. During transport or activities outside the patient's room, a portable oxygen tank is necessary. Check the portable tank to ensure an adequate supply is available. A nurse or respiratory therapist can set the oxygen flow for 2L. To transport the patient, unplug the oxygen tubing from the primary oxygen source, and plug it into the portable tank.

When placing your patient on the oxygen supply in his room, the color of the port that the oxygen tubing should be plugged into is:

Green

Rationale: The oxygen port available in a patient's room is green. When connecting the patient's oxygen tubing to the wall, be sure to plug the tubing into the green port. There may be other ports available, but the oxygen port is always green and labeled as oxygen.

Your patient has a pulse oximetry level of 82%. As a nursing assistant you should:

Notify the nurse

Rationale: A normal reading for a pulse oximetry is over 95%. Any reading under 95% is considered abnormal, and the nurse should be notified. This level may vary slightly depending on the patient's medical history, but the nurse will determine what action to take.

You are caring for a patient who is critically ill and is having shortness of breath. The oxygen saturation level is 69%. The nurse instructs you to call the respiratory therapist while she stays with the patient. The oxygen device used in a medical emergency is a:

Non-rebreather mask

Rationale: A non-rebreather mask is the best way to administer oxygen to a patient in an emergency situation. A non-rebreather mask covers the nose and mouth and provides the highest concentration of oxygen to a patient who is able to breathe unassisted. When placed properly, a non-rebreather mask can deliver 100% oxygen to a patient.

A patient receiving oxygen at 2L per minute by nasal cannula wants to go outside to smoke. The first thing that you should do is:

Inform the patient that oxygen is highly flammable, and then inform the nurse

Rationale: Oxygen is highly flammable, and the patient should always be educated about the hazards involved with its use. An open flame should never be allowed around oxygen, for the safety of the patient and the people around them. There are situations in which patients will demand to smoke, even after being educated about the dangers. The CNA should always inform the nurse when there are concerns that a patient may go outside to smoke, especially when he is on oxygen. The nurse and physician will determine how to handle the situation with the patient. Never remove oxygen from a patient without direction from the nurse, as this could cause his oxygen saturation to drop.

When having trouble getting an oxygen saturation reading by pulse oximeter on a patient's finger, you should:

Try to get the reading at a different site

Rationale: The finger is the most common site to obtain a reading but there are other options when unable to get an accurate reading. When unable to get a reading, first check for good contact. The finger should be clean, without nail polish or an artificial nail. The finger should be warm. If it's cold to the touch, the reading will be inaccurate. Other sites for a reading are the earlobe, toes, or nose.

A patient who wears a continuous nasal cannula complains of pain around her ears. On observation, you notice the skin is reddened. The first thing that you should do is:

Place padding around the tubing and notify the nurse

Rationale: Placing padding on the tubing by the ears will make the patient more comfortable, and to prevent skin breakdown. It is appropriate for the CNA to place padding around the oxygen tubing to provide comfort to the patient, and to prevent further skin breakdown. The most common sites to observe on a patient with a nasal cannula are over the ears, on the cheeks, under the nose, and under the chin.

----- COURSE TEST -----

1. What is a non-invasive procedure that measures the oxygen saturation of arterial blood?

A. Blood pressure

B. Pulse oximetry

C. Heart rate

D. ABG

XXXXXBXXXXX

2. What is a plastic device that administers oxygen through two prongs that are inserted into the nostrils?

A. Non-rebreather mask

B. Venturi mask

C. IV

D. Nasal cannula

XXXXXDXXXXX

3. What is an artificial opening into the trachea?

A. Tracheostomy

B. Iliostomy

C. Nasal cannula

D. Non-rebreather mask

XXXXXAXXXXX

4. You are caring for a patient who is on oxygen, which is being administered at 2L per minute by nasal cannula. When transporting the patient to the cafeteria for dinner, you should:

A. Remove the oxygen for dinner

B. Place the patient on a portable tank at 2L per minute

C. Change the oxygen setting to the maximum level

D. Take the oxygen off because you won't be long in the cafeteria

XXXXXBXXXXX

5. When connecting your patient to the oxygen supply in her room, what color port should the oxygen tubing be plugged into?

A. Red

B. Yellow

C. Blue

D. Green

XXXXXDXXXXX

6. Your patient has a pulse ox level of 82%. What should you do?

A. Notify the nurse

B. Recheck the level in fifteen minutes

C. Do nothing, this is a normal reading

D. Get the patient up and recheck the level after he walks around

XXXXXAXXXXX

7. You are caring for a patient who is critically ill and is having shortness of breath. The oxygen saturation level is 69%. The nurse instructs you to call the respiratory therapist while she stays with the patient. What is the oxygen device used in a medical emergency?

A. Nasal cannula

B. Venturi mask

C. Non-rebreather mask

D. Oxygen tent

XXXXXCXXXXX

8. What is the first thing you should do if your patient who is receiving oxygen at 2L per minute by nasal cannula wants to go outside to smoke?

A. Inform the patient that oxygen is highly flammable, and then inform the nurse

B. Let him go outside to smoke

C. Put him on a portable oxygen tank

D. Take the oxygen off

XXXXXAXXXXX

9. When having trouble getting an oxygen saturation reading by pulse oximeter reading on a patient's finger, you should?

A. Record what the last pulse ox reading was

B. Try to get the pulse ox reading later

C. Try to get the reading at a different site

D. Tell the nurse that you are unable to obtain the reading

XXXXXCXXXXX

10. A patient who wears a continuous nasal cannula complains of pain around her ears. On observation, you notice the skin is reddened. What is the first thing that you should do?

A. Remove the oxygen tubing

B. Place padding around the tubing and notify the nurse

C. Switch the patient to another form of oxygen administration

D. Do nothing, as this is a common problem when wearing oxygen

XXXXXBXXXXX

COURSE # 26 - Sensory Perceptions & Impairments

A 29-year-old female who was blinded in a car accident asks for help walking to the bathroom for the first time. You should:

Walk in front of the patient with the patient's hand on your elbow.

Rationale: The walking companion should precede the patient by about one foot, with the patient's hand on the guide's elbow to provide security. The guide should give short, concise directions about steps, inclines, turns, or obstacles.

A hearing-impaired patient has problems communicating with staff members. It might not help to:

Speak loudly

Rationale: Speaking loudly does not overcome communication difficulties with hearing-impaired people. It can also violate a patient's right to privacy. Get the patient's attention by raising your hand or touching him gently, then speak in conversational tones while facing him or speak directly into the less-affected ear. Some hearing deficiencies are tone-based, with higher pitched sounds being difficult to hear. Try speaking with a deeper voice. If this technique is successful, document it for other staff members.

Myopia is a medical term for the visual disorder of:

Nearsightedness

Rationale: Myopia means being able to clearly see objects that are near. Objects in the distance appear fuzzy or blurry. In order to see things far away, eyeglasses or contact lenses are necessary.

When caring for a patient who is blind or visually impaired, it is important to:

Announce when you enter and leave the room

Rationale: You should introduce yourself each time you enter the room until the patient recognizes your voice. Always speak to the patient, telling her what you plan to do. Be sure to describe what is on a plate or tray and tell the patient where each item is located, using a clock as a reference. It is appropriate to say goodbye with a tap on the person's arm. Voice tone should be pleasant and friendly.

Astigmatism is a medical term for:

Blurred vision

Rationale: Astigmatism refers to a vision defect that causes blurred vision. Due to the irregular eye surface, light enters the lens in an uneven way, causing objects to look fuzzy. Astigmatism is common, and easily corrected by eyeglasses, contact lenses, or surgery.

Conjunctivitis is commonly called:

Pinkeye

Rationale: Conjunctivitis, commonly known as pinkeye, is an inflammation of the conjunctiva, the clear membrane that covers the white part of the eye and the inner surface of the eyelids. Causes include bacterial or viral infection, allergy, or environmental factors. Symptoms include itching, burning, stinging, irritation, pain, grittiness, crusting, or light sensitivity. Conjunctivitis is extremely contagious. Poor hand washing is the main reason for spread of pinkeye.

A diabetic patient has severe neuropathy in his feet. As a CNA, you should be alert for:

Foot injuries

Rationale: One of the complications of diabetes is neuropathy, a loss of sensation. Without the ability to feel, a patient may suffer an injury and not know it. When performing care, healthcare staff should check a diabetic patient's feet for redness, cuts, bruises, or blisters. Footwear and socks that are too tight may also cause decreased circulation.

An early sign of age-related hearing loss is:

Difficulty understanding conversation in public places

Rationale: Age-related hearing loss is a gradual process. Elderly people may turn up the television volume, not be able to hear women and children, or have difficulty understanding conversation in public or noisy places. Healthcare workers or family may notice the hearing loss first. A hearing evaluation is indicated to determine if a hearing aid may be useful.

In orienting a visually-impaired patient to a meal, the CNA would:

Identify food according to an imaginary clock face

Rationale: Describe the contents of the meal. You can either use the clock-face method, e.g. the meat is at six o'clock, or by saying items are at the top, bottom, right or left side of the plate. Meat should be placed at six o'clock, for easy cutting. Color contrast can be important for people who are visually-impaired. Placing a dark tray or cloth under a light plate defines the plate edges, making it easier to locate the food. Ask the patient if he needs "assistance with his meal" rather than offering to "cut up his food."

When caring for a patient who has difficulty speaking, it is appropriate to:

Use a communication board

Rationale: Communication boards provide a visual way for a patient to communicate with staff, family, and visitors. These low-technology displays consist of photographs, symbols, words, phrases, or a combination of all three.

----- COURSE TEST -----

1. When a 29-year-old female who was blinded in a car accident asks for help walking to the bathroom for the first time, what should you do?

A. Walk in front of the patient with the patient's hand on your elbow

B. Walk behind the patient with the patient's hand on your elbow

C. Walk in front of the patient and notify her of any obstacles in her path

D. Walk behind the patient with your hand on her shoulder

XXXXXAXXXXX

2. A hearing-impaired patient has problems communicating with staff members. Which behavior would be least helpful?

A. Speaking loudly

B. Facing the patient when speaking

C. Speaking in conversational tones

D. Speaking into the less-affected ear

XXXXXAXXXXX

3. Myopia is a medical term meaning which visual disorder?

A. Farsightedness

B. Blurry vision

C. Nearsightedness

D. Spotted vision

XXXXXCXXXXX

4. What is important when caring for a patient who is blind or visually impaired?

A. Keeping all items within the person's reach

B. Color coding all important paperwork

C. Announcing when you enter and leave the room

D. Placing all furniture up against the walls

XXXXXCXXXXX

5. Astigmatism is a medical term that means?

A. Blurred vision

B. Inability to detect colors

C. Color blindness

D. Farsightedness

XXXXXAXXXXX

6. What is conjunctivitis more commonly called?

A. An infection

B. Tearing

C. Pink eye

D. Color blindness

XXXXXCXXXXX

7. A diabetic patient has severe neuropathy in his feet. What should a CNA check for?

A. Changes in walking

B. Foot injuries

C. Ability to put on shoes

D. Bunions

XXXXXBXXXXX

8. An early sign of age-related hearing loss is?

A. Listening to songs from high school

B. Ignoring a spouse during a family visit

C. Difficulty understanding conversation in public places

D. Whispering to the CNA during a bed bath

XXXXXCXXXXX

9. How would the CNA help in orienting a visually impaired patient to a meal?

A. Identify the location of the plate

B. Hold the patient's hand and direct it to the plate

C. Put the eating utensil in the patient's hand

D. Identify food according to an imaginary clock face

XXXXXDXXXXX

10. When caring for a patient who has difficulty speaking, what is an appropriate action?

A. Call for an interpreter

B. Use a communication board

C. Communicate through family members

D. Ask the patient to write everything down

XXXXXBXXXXX

COURSE # 27 - Stages of Grief

The deep feeling of sorrow following a loss is called:

Grief

Rationale: Grief is a normal response to loss. While grief is a natural reaction to a loved one's death, other losses can cause sadness. The death of a pet can be a painful experience. People who work in healthcare may grieve the death of a special patient. Grief is a universal experience, but how people express grief depends on each individual, as well as the individual's culture.

The expression of grief following a loss is:

Mourning

Rationale: Mourning is an external response to a loss. It has been described as how we show grief in public. Mourning is influenced by culture, religious beliefs, and family customs. Examples of mourning include wearing black or bringing flowers to the grave on special days.

The period of time after a loss when grief and mourning occur is:

Bereavement

Rationale: The length of time for bereavement is different for each person. The process involves emotional, social, and physical adjustment to the loss. Factors affecting bereavement include how close the deceased person was, circumstances of the death, and the support system in place to ease the loss. Bereavement is one of the most difficult times in a person's life. It takes time and effort, and the process should be respected by others.

A therapy used to help a person after a loss or a death by talking and expressing feelings related to the loss is:

Grief counseling

Rationale: Grief counseling is an option that can be useful following a loss. By expressing feelings and working through initial steps of living without the loved one, healing can take place. Grief counseling may be private or in a group setting.

It is important to allow family members to stay with a dying family member:

As often as possible

Rationale: The dying process is a stressful and sad time for family members. It is important for the family members to feel that they are welcome at any time, and that they can be part of the team. Many hospitals provide beds and kitchen facilities for family members.

Denial, anger, bargaining, and depression are four of the five stages of grief. The fifth stage is:

Acceptance

Rationale: The theory of the five stages of grief was first introduced by Dr. Elisabeth Kubler-Ross in 1969. Her theory was based on her observations and conversations with terminally ill patients. She called the final stage acceptance. This is when a person comes to terms with the loss and is able to accept the outcome. The five stages represent feelings and emotions of going through a loss. Each person progresses at a different pace, often moving back and forth between the stages.

The first stage of the grieving process is:

Denial

Rationale: Denial is the initial reaction to a loss. The first word spoken is "No." People can't believe what has happened; they think there has been a mistake or mix-up. News of the loss seems impossible. Denial includes a state of shock; people are unable to listen to information or make decisions. The CNA can provide support and comfort during this stage. Offer a quiet place to sit, something to drink, and access to a phone.

The stage of grief in which a person tries to make deals to gain extra time or to make amends is:

Bargaining

Rationale: Bargaining is the stage when people understand that there is a loss, but hope to delay the ending. A patient may pray for time to attend a family event or promise to do something in return for a cure or a different outcome. People often feel guilty for past actions or behaviors, and try to negotiate for a chance to make amends before dying or moving on to something new.

The length of time that it takes to move through the stages of grief is:

Different for each person

Rationale: There is no timeline for any loss. Factors such as the type of loss and its personal meaning, available support systems, and religious and cultural beliefs will affect the grieving process. The stages of grief are not rigid. A person can move back and forth among the stages many times. One day may be easy, the next will be difficult. Always treat a grieving person with patience and respect.

When giving support to a grieving person, you should:

Listen with compassion

Rationale: As a CNA, you may frequently have the opportunity to comfort family members and co-workers who are experiencing a loss. It is important to listen with compassion and to acknowledge that everyone grieves in different ways. Accept their feelings and emotions, and understand that grief has no timeline.

----- COURSE TEST -----

1. What is the deep feeling of sorrow following a loss called?

A. Fear

B. Grief

C. Anger

D. Compassion

XXXXXBXXXXX

2. The expression of grief following a loss is called?

A. Fear

B. Grief

C. Mourning

D. Loss

XXXXXCXXXXX

3. What is the period of time after a loss when grief and mourning occur?

A. Bereavement

B. Grief

C. Loss

D. Anger

XXXXXAXXXXX

4. What is a therapy called that is often used after a loss or a death that may help a person through talking and expressing feelings?

A. Depression

B. Life regression

C. Hypnosis

D. Grief counseling

XXXXXDXXXXX

5. How often should family members be allowed to stay with a dying patient?

A. Once per day

B. During visiting hours

C. As often as possible

D. Only when the patient is awake

XXXXXCXXXXX

6. Denial, anger, bargaining, and depression are four of the five stages of grief. What is the fifth stage?

A. Recovery

B. Acceptance

C. Depression

D. Loss

XXXXXBXXXXX

7. What is the first stage of the grieving process?

A. Denial

B. Loss

C. Acceptance

D. Recovery

XXXXXAXXXXX

8. What is the stage of grief called in which a person tries to make deals to gain extra time or to make amends?

A. Depression

B. Acceptance

C. Denial

D. Bargaining

XXXXXDXXXXX

9. What is the length of time that a person will spend in the stages of grief?

A. It differs for each person

B. One year

C. Three days

D. One month

XXXXXAXXXXX

10. What is an important step when supporting a grieving person?

A. Encourage him to spend time alone

B. Listen with compassion

C. Never allow him to talk about the death

D. Place little value on his feelings since he is grieving

XXXXXBXXXXX

COURSE # 28 - Stress Management

A condition in which the body responds to any changes from its normal balanced state is:

Stress

Rationale: Stress is normal, and it can have both positive and negative effects. These effects are physical, emotional, intellectual, social, and spiritual. Positive stress can be energizing and motivating. Negative stress can affect health, emotions, and relationships. A career as a CNA involves daily stress. Learning stress management techniques is important both personally and professionally.

Anything causing stress is called:

A stressor

Rationale: A stressor is anything that causes stress, either internal or external. Internal stressors include things such as feeling ill or having menstrual cycle cramps. External stressors happen outside the body. Examples are having a heavy patient load, financial worries, or dealing with a critical supervisor.

Stress can be reduced through:

Regular exercise

Rationale: The benefits of regular exercise include improving your physical health through cardiovascular conditioning, weight control, and improved blood pressure. Exercise also relieves tension and promotes relaxation. General health guidelines suggest 30 to 45 minutes of exercise three to four times per week.

Optimal health and body function depends on:

Nutrition

Rationale: Proper nutrition is essential in maintaining health and dealing with stress. Poor eating habits contribute to obesity, diabetes, and high blood pressure. By eating a balanced diet, and avoiding junk food, internal stress is reduced. Good nutrition provides more energy to enjoy life.

Specific methods to deal with stress, such as relaxation and meditation, are examples of:

Stress management techniques

Rationale: Stress management techniques are methods of dealing with the physical and emotional consequences of stress. Along with regular exercise, other ways to reduce or control stress include yoga, meditation, or deep breathing. Hobbies, crafts, sports, and time with family or friends are natural stress reducers. Managing stress improves both mental outlook and quality of life.

Home care of family members for long periods of time may cause chronic stress called:

Caregiver burnout

Rationale: Caregiver burnout is chronic stress that can have a major impact on family members who provide care to loved ones. Common symptoms include depression, fatigue, sleep problems, and even physical illnesses such as high blood pressure, and heart disease. As CNAs, it is important to watch for these behaviors when caring for patients and families, and to provide support when possible.

Laughing and crying are two examples of unconsciously dealing with anxiety. These are called:

Coping mechanisms

Rationale: Coping mechanisms are individual ways people automatically deal with stress. Behaviors such as crying, laughing, cursing, and lack of eye contact are all examples of coping mechanisms.

When coping mechanisms are not adequate for reducing stress, other behaviors are used which are called:

Defense mechanisms

Rationale: Defense mechanisms are used to protect one's self-esteem and are used for all types of stress. Some examples are compensation (making up for a sense of inadequacy, such as boasting), rationalization (creating reasons to justify a thought or action), and denial (refusal to face or accept reality). Defense mechanisms can be observed in our patients, as well as in ourselves and co-workers.

A patient who refuses to acknowledge the presence of a disease may be using a defensive mechanism called:

Denial

Rationale: Denial is a common defense mechanism that may be seen in a patient when she is having trouble dealing with stress in her life, such as diagnosis of a disease. Denial serves as a temporary shock-absorber, allowing the patient time to face the situation.

When coping and defense mechanisms are no longer effective, it is called a:

Crisis

Rationale: A crisis is the result of loss of self-esteem from events such as illness, sense of failure, or complete loss of control. A person in a crisis situation needs immediate help, and his behavior should never be ignored. A CNA should be aware of crisis behaviors, such as high levels of anxiety, disorganized behavior, and inability to function as usual. A CNA may be the first person on the healthcare team to recognize a patient in a crisis. Always report unusual behavior to the nurse.

----- COURSE TEST -----

1. What is a condition in which the body responds to any change from its normally balanced state?

A. Reflex

B. Inflammation

C. Stress

D. Habits

XXXXXCXXXXX

2. What is anything that causes a person to experience stress?

A. Stressor

B. Coping

C. Death

D. Grief

XXXXXAXXXXX

3. What can reduce stress?

A. Smoking

B. Regular exercise

C. Talking

D. Drinking alcohol

XXXXXBXXXXX

4. What maintains optimal health and body function?

A. Crisis

B. Stressors

C. Working overtime

D. Nutrition

XXXXXDXXXXX

5. What are methods, such as relaxation and meditation, that help us deal with stress?

A. Stress management techniques

B. Crisis intervention

C. Support system

D. Adaptation

XXXXXAXXXXX

6. What is the chronic stress experienced by family members who provide home care?

A. Crisis

B. Caregiver burnout

C. Anxiety

D. Defense mechanism

XXXXXBXXXXX

7. What are subconscious ways of dealing with mild anxiety?

A. Stressors

B. Anxiety

C. Adaptation

D. Coping mechanisms

XXXXXDXXXXX

8. What is a mechanism used to deal with stress when coping mechanisms are not adequate?

A. Defense mechanism

B. Prolonged stress

C. Mind-body interaction

D. Adaptation

XXXXXAXXXXX

9. What is a defense mechanism in which a patient refuses to acknowledge the presence of a disease?

A. Projection

B. Compensation

C. Denial

D. Suppression

XXXXXCXXXXX

10. What is a situation in which coping and defense mechanisms are no longer effective?

A. Crisis

B. Reactions

C. Depression

D. Anxiety

XXXXXAXXXXX

COURSE # 29 - Vital Signs

The least accurate method of assessing body temperature is:

Axillary

Rationale: Axillary temperatures are taken by putting a thermometer under the armpit for four to five minutes. Because the armpit does not provide the temperature of the body core, the reading will be about two degrees lower than a rectal temperature.

Difficulty in breathing is called:

Dyspnea

Rationale: Dyspnea, shortness of breath (SOB), or air hunger, is difficulty breathing. It can be the result of disease, such as emphysema or asthma, or natural activity, such as running or exercise.

Korotkoff sounds are heard when taking a patient's:

Blood pressure

Rationale: Korotkoff sounds are used to determine blood pressure when using a stethoscope and blood pressure cuff. The first sound heard after releasing the cuff is the systolic blood pressure number. The last sound is the diastolic blood pressure number.

One full count of a respiration includes:

An inspiration and expiration

Rationale: One respiratory cycle includes one full inspiration and one complete expiration. The volume of air that enters or leaves during a single respiratory cycle is called the tidal volume. Tidal volume is typically 500 milliliters, meaning that 500 milliliters of air enters during inspiration and the same amount leaves during expiration.

The normal temperature of an adult is:

98.6 F

Rationale: Normal human body core temperature is 98.6°F, or 37°C. Normal temperatures vary with the time of day and with the type of exercise. Normal temperature ranges are different for infants, children, and adults.

The most common site for taking a pulse is the:

Radial artery

Rationale: There are several sites on the body where a pulse is normally taken. All arteries have a pulse, but it is easier to palpate (feel) the pulse at certain locations. It is easier to feel the pulse when the artery is near the surface of the skin and when there is firm tissue (such as a bone) beneath the artery. The two most common sites are the radial (wrist) and carotid (throat).

A healthy heart rate for an adult is:

60-80 beats per minute (bpm)

Rationale: For healthy adults, a lower heart rate at rest generally implies more efficient heart function and better cardiovascular fitness. Heart rate can be affected by activity and fitness levels, body position (standing, sitting, or lying), emotional state, body size, and medication use. External factors, such as temperature and humidity, can also affect heart rate.

An abbreviation for vital signs is:

TPR

Rationale: TPR stands for Temperature, Pulse, and Respiration. In many health care settings, TPR is recorded as part of a routine shift or doctor visit.

This blood pressure reading may indicate hypertension:

140/90

Rationale: A single high blood pressure reading does not necessarily mean that a patient has hypertension (high blood pressure). If blood pressure remains elevated over several readings and under normal circumstances, the doctor may start treatment. Hypertension is treated with diet, exercise, and medication.

A way to determine how much pain a patient is experiencing is to use a:

Pain scale

Rationale: Pain is subjective; the only person who can describe the level of discomfort is the patient. When assessing pain, ask a patient to tell how much pain he is experiencing on a scale of one to ten, with ten being the highest. Pain scales are also available as pictures of faces, from smiling (level one) to grimacing (level ten).

----- COURSE TEST -----

1. What is the least accurate method of assessing body temperature?

A. Oral

B. Rectal

C. Axillary

D. Tympanic

XXXXXCXXXXX

2. What it is called when a patient has difficulty breathing?

A. Orthopnea

B. Dyspnea

C. Apnea

D. Cheyne-Stokes respirations

XXXXXBXXXXX

3. What sounds are heard when taking a blood pressure?

A. Korotkoff sounds

B. Respirations

C. Valve murmurs

D. Heart rate

XXXXXAXXXXX

4. What does one full count of respiration include?

A. Two inspirations and expirations

B. One inspiration

C. One expiration

D. An inspiration and expiration

XXXXXDXXXXX

5. What is the normal temperature of an adult?

A. 100.6 F

B. 99 F

C. 98.6 F

D. 96.8 F

XXXXXCXXXXX

6. What is the most common site for taking a pulse?

A. Radial artery

B. Brachial artery

C. Carotid artery

D. Dorsalis pedis artery

XXXXXAXXXXX

7. What is a healthy heart rate for an adult?

A. 40-60 bpm

B. 60-80 bpm

C. 80-100 bpm

D. 100-120 bpm

XXXXXBXXXXX

8. What is the abbreviation for vital signs?

A. ROM

B. TPR

C. BID

D. QID

XXXXXBXXXXX

9. After several blood pressure checks, which indicates hypertension?

A. 100/60

B. 120/80

C. 140/90

D. Depends on several factors

XXXXXCXXXXX

What is one way to determine how much pain a patient is experiencing?

A. A pain formula

B. A pain scale

C. Pain medication

D. Pain management

XXXXXBXXXXX

COURSE # 30 - Vital Signs 2

A patient with a pulse that is slower than normal has a condition called:

Bradycardia

Rationale: The average pulse for adults is 60-80 beats per minute. A heart rate that is lower than normal for a patient is called bradycardia. The cause may be a problem with the electrical pathways in the heart, or with the heart's natural "pacemaker." When the heart beats at a slow rate, oxygen saturation levels drop. Bradycardia is an emergency and should be reported to the nurse.

When taking blood pressure, the first number that is recorded is called:

Systolic pressure

Rationale: Blood pressure is recorded as two numbers, the systolic and diastolic pressures. The first, and higher, number (systolic pressure) is the measurement of the pressure against the arterial walls when the heart beats. The second, and lower, number is the pressure against the arterial walls while the heart rests between heart beats.

As death nears, the breathing pattern changes to what is called:

Cheyne-Stokes

Rationale: One of the signs of approaching death is Cheyne-Stokes breathing. The patient will take deep rapid breaths, followed by shallow breaths, then stop breathing (apnea) for a short time. The cycle repeats, with the periods of apnea growing longer. This pattern is normal for the end of life. The CNA can explain Cheyne-Stokes to the family and provide support during this time.

The vital sign that is difficult to quantify because it relies on input from the patient is called:

Pain

Rationale: Assessment of pain is an important part of patient care and treatment. Pain is subjective; only the patient can determine the level of pain. When a patient is conscious and alert, a pain scale can be used. The patient is asked to report his pain on a scale of one to ten, with ten being the worst possible. Healthcare workers should not decide for or judge a patient's self-assessment of pain. When a patient is unconscious or non-verbal, pain can be assessed by facial expression, clenched teeth, crying, restlessness, or increased blood pressure and pulse.

The healthcare workers responsible for making adjustments to a patient's ventilator are called:

Respiratory therapists

Rationale: When a patient is intubated, respiratory therapists are responsible for following the physician's orders to make the adjustments to the ventilator. The ventilator controls the respiratory rate and oxygen saturation level. Respiratory therapists also provide breathing treatments and monitor supplemental oxygen for patients who are not intubated.

While taking a patient's blood pressure, you notice that it is unusually lower than normal. This situation is called:

Hypotension

Rationale: Normal blood pressure is 120/80. A reading of 90/60 or lower is considered to be hypotension. Hypotension may be caused by dehydration, medications such as water pills (diuretics) or blood pressure medications, a low heart rate (bradycardia), or remaining in the same position for a long time. Severe hypotension can also be a symptom of shock, a medical emergency. Report hypotension to the nurse for further evaluation.

The display of the heart's electrical activity called an:

ECG

Rationale: The electrocardiogram, ECG or EKG, is a non-invasive test used to measure the electrical activity of the heart. Electrodes (leads) are placed at specific spots on the chest. When connected to the ECG machine, the heart's electrical activity is displayed on a monitor or printed out. The ECG is analyzed for the heart rate; for the consistency and strength of electrical activity; and for irregular patterns. An ECG can show if a heart attack is occurring or occurred in the past, if there are problems with the heart valves, if the heart is beating irregularly, or if heart failure is present. After reading an abnormal ECG, physicians can determine the best treatment for the patient.

The medical term for profuse sweating is called:

Diaphoresis

Rationale: Excessive sweating is called diaphoresis. The most common cause is an elevated temperature, or fever, from an illness. Other causes include a heart attack, alcohol withdrawal, menopause, and all types of shock. Anxiety, pain, heat exhaustion, and motion sickness can cause diaphoresis outside the healthcare setting. Exercise and being in warm temperatures also cause heavy sweating. Diaphoresis is automatic, and is the result of the body trying to cool off.

Examining a patient through the use of touch is called:

Palpation

Rationale: Palpation is using the hands and fingers to assess a patient. By using touch, a physician can check the size, shape, texture, consistency, and firmness of an internal organ or an area of the body. Palpation helps in diagnosing a disease, in locating the source of pain, or assessing a condition, such as swelling in the legs (edema).

If a patient's pulse cannot be found by touch or auscultation (listening with a stethoscope), the alternative method used is called:

Doppler ultrasound

Rationale: With certain patient conditions, it can be difficult to find a pulse through touch, especially during code and trauma situations. A Doppler device can be used at the bedside to locate and record a pulse. Gel is applied to the device and the Doppler is placed at the area of the pulse. Even a faint sound can be heard with a Doppler, showing that blood is circulating.

----- COURSE TEST -----

1. A patient with a pulse that is slower than normal has a condition called?

A. Bradycardia

B. Tachycardia

C. Bradypnea

D. Tachypnea

XXXXXAXXXXX

2. What is the reading that refers to the blood being pushed into the arterial network by the heart called when taking blood pressure?

A. Diastolic pressure

B. Cardiac pressure

C. Coronary pressure

D. Systolic pressure

XXXXXDXXXXX

3. What is the breathing pattern observed at the end of life?

A. Kussmaul

B. Cheyne-Stokes

C. Hyperventilation

D. Paroxysmal Dyspnea

XXXXXBXXXXX

4. What is the vital sign that is difficult to quantify because it relies on input from the patient?

A. Blood pressure

B. Heart rate

C. Pain

D. Respiratory rate

XXXXXCXXXXX

5. Who are the healthcare workers responsible for making adjustments to a patient's ventilator?

A. Radiologic Technologists

B. Respiratory Therapists

C. Nurses

D. Certified Nursing Aides

XXXXXBXXXXX

6. While taking a patient's blood pressure, you notice that it is unusually lower than normal. What is this situation called?

A. Bradycardia

B. Hypertension

C. Hypotension

D. Tachypnea

XXXXXCXXXXX

7. What is the medical test used to measure the electrical activity of the heart called?

A. Sphygmomanometer

B. Blood pressure cuff

C. Pulse oximeter

D. Electrocardiogram

XXXXXDXXXXX

8. What is the medical term used for profuse sweating?

A. Cyanosis

B. Diaphoresis

C. Tachyaresis

D. Autonomia nevosus

XXXXXBXXXXX

9. What is the examining of a patient through the use of touch called?

A. Palpitation

B. Palpation

C. Caressing

D. Addressing

XXXXXBXXXXX

10. If a patient's pulse cannot be found by touch or auscultation (listening with a stethoscope) what method can be used?

A. Chest radiography

B. CT Scan

C. Doppler ultrasound

D. PET ultrasound

XXXXXCXXXXX

COURSE # 31 - Vital Signs 3

The ECG reading of a flat line indicates:

Asystole

Rationale: When the heart is not producing any electrical activity, the ECG/EKG reading produces a flat line. Asystole means that the heart is not beating, so no blood is circulating. There will be no blood pressure. A Code Blue is called for asystole; CPR is given until the code team arrives. After several minutes of asystole, a physician can declare a patient dead.

A positive leukocyte reading in a urinalysis can help confirm:

Urinary tract infections

Rationale: Leukocytes are white blood cells that fight an infection. They travel to the site of the infection or injury. If a urinalysis (UA) is positive for leukocytes, a physician can diagnose a urinary tract infection (UTI) and prescribe antibiotics. Patients with a UTI may complain of pain or burning when urinating, frequent urination, or the urge to urinate but little or no output. A CNA may notice that the urine is cloudy, red, or bright pink, and strong-smelling. Report any of these signs or symptoms to the nurse.

A rectal temperature reading is higher than an oral reading by:

.5 to 1 degree Fahrenheit

Rationale: There are four ways to take a temperature. Normal oral temperature for an adult is 98.6 degrees Fahrenheit. The oral method is appropriate for adults and older children. Rectal temperatures are .5 to 1 degree higher than oral. Rectal temperatures are the most accurate; this is the preferred method for babies. Tympanic (ear) temperatures are also 5. to 1 degree higher than oral; this method can be used for all ages. Axillary (armpit) temperatures are about .5 to 1 degree lower than oral. This method is appropriate for all ages, especially older patients. All methods can provide an accurate temperature when done correctly.

The heart rate of 105 bpm is considered:

Tachycardic

Rationale: Depending on age and physical condition, the normal range for an adult resting heart rate is 60-100 beats per minute (bpm). Tachycardia is a resting heart rate is above 100 bpm. Tachycardia results from abnormal electrical activity in the upper chambers of the heart. The heart beats so rapidly that blood doesn't have time to fill the chambers and circulation is poor. A patient may feel dizzy or light-headed. Because less oxygen is circulated, the patient may experience shortness of breath or chest pain. The CNA should report a pulse of greater than 100 bpm to the nurse.

The blood pressure reading of 130/85 is considered:

Pre-hypertension

Rationale: A blood pressure between 120/80 and 139/89 is considered to be pre-hypertensive. This means there is a risk of developing high blood pressure (hypertension) in the future. Lifestyle changes can control pre-hypertension and prevent hypertension. Exercise, diet, weight control, and not smoking will lower the risk of stroke, heart disease, kidney disease, and dementia.

The medical term for a fever is called:

Pyrexia

Rationale: A fever (pyrexia) is a rise in temperature as the body responds to an illness or infection. Pyrexia is a natural way of fighting bacteria and viruses. Normal body temperature is 98.6 degrees Fahrenheit. A fever is a temperature of 100.4 degrees or higher.
A patient with a fever may experience chills, shivering, sweating, headache, stiff muscles, and loss of appetite. The CNA can offer frequent liquids to prevent dehydration.

The second level of consciousness is:

Drowsy but responsive

Rationale: There are four levels of consciousness (LOC). The first LOC is alert and conscious. The patient is aware of his surroundings and can answer questions accurately. The second LOC is drowsy but responsive. The patient may be extremely lethargic, but will answer questions slowly or after a delay. The third LOC is unconscious but responsive to painful stimulation. The patient is nonverbal, possibly unconscious, but reacts to pain. The fourth LOC is comatose. The patient is completely incapacitated and does not respond to questioning or stimulus of any kind.

A normal respiratory rate for an adult is:

Twelve to twenty breaths per minute

Rationale: A healthy adult will breathe at a rate of twelve to twenty breaths per minute. To record the respirations per minute, just count the number of inhalations the patient makes in a sixty second period.

A patient with low blood oxygen levels is diagnosed with:

Hypoxemia

Rationale: Oxygen saturation, or O2 sat, is the percentage of oxygen in the blood. The normal O2 sat range is 95-100%. Patients with lung disease may have a normal O2 sat level. Any drop in O2 sat requires intervention. The physician may order supplemental oxygen to bring the level up to what is normal for the patient. In a hospital, respiratory therapists will be responsible for monitoring the patient's oxygen saturation. The CNA may be asked to record the O2 sat readings from the pulse oximeter.

An hCG test is also known as a:

Pregnancy test

Rationale: An hCG test is the most accurate way to diagnose pregnancy. hCG (HCG), human chorionic gonadotropin, is the hormone produced by the placenta. An hCG blood test can detect pregnancy ten days after conception. An hCG urine test will show results fourteen days after conception. In a healthcare setting, hCG testing may be ordered on any female patient over age ten. This is a routine precautionary test, intended to protect an unborn baby before treatment is given.

----- COURSE TEST -----

1. What does the ECG reading of a flat line indicate?

A. Asystole

B. Asepsis

C. Apneic

D. Apical

XXXXXAXXXXX

2. What can a positive leukocyte reading in a urinalysis help confirm?

A. High protein levels in blood

B. Urinary tract infections

C. URI

D. Blood in the urine

XXXXXBXXXXX

3. How much higher than oral are rectally taken temperatures?

A. .5 to 1 degrees Fahrenheit

B. 1 to 2 degrees Fahrenheit

C. 1.5 degrees Fahrenheit

D. Trick question, it is .5 to 1 degrees Fahrenheit cooler

XXXXXAXXXXX

4. What is the heart rate 105 bpm considered?

A. Normal

B. Slightly elevated

C. Bradycardic

D. Tachycardic

XXXXXDXXXXX

5. What is a blood pressure reading of 130/85-considered?

A. Pre-hypertension

B. Normal

C. Stage 1 hypertension

D. Stage 2 hypertension

XXXXXAXXXXX

6. What is the medical term for a fever?

A. Pyroxia

B. Pyromania

C. Pyrexia

D. Pyremia

XXXXXCXXXXX

7. What is the second level of consciousness?

A. Comatose

B. Alert and conscious

C. Responsive to painful stimuli

D. Drowsy but responsive

XXXXXDXXXXX

8. What is the normal respiratory rate for an adult?

A. Sixteen to twenty breaths per minute

B. Ten to twenty breaths per minute

C. Twelve to twenty breaths per minute

D. Twelve to sixteen breaths per minute

XXXXXCXXXXX

9. What is a patient with low blood oxygen levels diagnosed with?

A. Hyperoxemia

B. Hypoxemia

C. Hypoemia

D. Hypovolemia

XXXXXBXXXXX

10. What is an hCG test also known as?

A. Blood test

B. Urine culture

C. Pregnancy test

D. Blood sugar test

XXXXXCXXXXX

COURSE # 32 - Vital Signs Overview

The normal pulse rate for an adult patient is:

60 to 100 bpm

Rationale: The normal pulse rate for an adult patient is 60 to 100 beats per minute (bpm). There are numerous factors that can influence heart rate, including age and medical history.

When obtaining a pulse on a patient, typically the easiest place to feel the pulse is the:

Radial artery

Rationale: The radial artery is found in the inside of the wrist, on the same side as the patient's thumb. Always feel this area with your first two fingers, and not your thumb (using your own thumb may cause you to feel your own pulse). The carotid (neck) artery is a good alternative for obtaining an accurate pulse.

The nurse asks you to obtain an apical pulse on a patient. This pulse is obtained by using:

A stethoscope

Rationale: An apical pulse is obtained using a stethoscope to listen to the pulse on the chest, directly over the heart. The apical pulse is the most accurate; it is the preferred method when a radial pulse can't be detected.

When taking vital signs on an adult patient and his respiratory rate is forty, he is sweating, and is complaining of mild pain, you should:

Tell the nurse immediately

Rationale: The normal respiratory rate for an adult is twelve to twenty breaths per minute. Always report any unusual vital signs or symptoms to the nurse.

When taking a blood pressure you should pump the blood pressure cuff:

30 mm Hg above the point at which the pulse disappears

Rationale: You should always listen for the pulse as you are taking the blood pressure. As you pump up the cuff, listen for the point where the pulse disappears, then inflate the cuff another 30 mm Hg.

The nurse requests that you get a rectal temperature on a patient. You should:

Use a designated thermometer with a red probe, inserted into the rectum

Rationale: A rectal temperature is obtained by inserting a designated probe into the rectum. These rectal thermometers typically have a red probe. Lubricate the thermometer before inserting into the rectum.

When attempting to obtain a blood pressure on an obese patient and the blood pressure cuff will not fit all the way around the patient's arm, you should:

Use a larger cuff

Rationale: An accurate blood pressure reading depends on a well-fitting cuff. Blood pressure cuffs have markings to ensure a proper fit. An obese patient will need a larger cuff. Blood pressure cuffs are simply screwed in to the blood pressure device; choose the cuff that fits the patient's arm for an accurate reading.

Your patient's blood pressure is 115/75. The upper number 115 represents:

The systolic pressure

Rationale: The top number on a blood pressure reading is the systolic pressure, which represents the highest amount of pressure on arterial walls while the heart is contracting. The bottom number is the diastolic pressure, which represents the least amount of pressure applied on the walls, which occurs while the heart is resting between contractions.

When you enter your patient's room to obtain a blood pressure and realize the patient has an IV infusing to the left arm, you should:

Take the blood pressure from the right arm

Rationale: When a patient has an IV, the blood pressure should be taken in the arm opposite the site of the IV. The pressure of inflating a cuff on the same side of an IV can stop the flow of fluid and medication being infused, and may allow the vein to clot from the pressure of the cuff inflation.

When counting the respiratory rate on your patient, it is important to:

Watch the rise and fall of the chest a minimum of thirty seconds

Rationale: It is important to watch the chest rise and fall to accurately count inspiration and expiration. This should be done for a minimum of thirty seconds, then multiply by two to calculate respirations for a minute. You should watch for a full minute if the respirations are irregular. It is recommended to count while you are taking the pulse, allowing the patient to speak normally so she continues to breathe as usual.

----- COURSE TEST -----

1. What is the normal pulse rate for an adult patient?

A. 60-100

B. 50-70

C. 80-100

D. 30-50

XXXXXAXXXXX

2. Typically, where is the easiest and most common place to feel the pulse on a patient?

A. Apical

B. Radial artery

C. Carotid artery

D. Femoral artery

XXXXXBXXXXX

3. What do you use when a nurse asks you to obtain an apical pulse on a patient?

A. A thermometer

B. A stethoscope

C. A blood pressure cuff

D. Your hand

XXXXXBXXXXX

4. What should do when you are taking vital signs on an adult patient whose respiratory rate is 40, and the patient is sweating and complaining of mild pain?

A. Nothing, the patient often complains of pain and this is common

B. Tell him to relax, and check on him after you are done getting vital signs on all of your patients

C. Tell the nurse immediately

D. Get him some water

XXXXXCXXXXX

5. When taking a blood pressure on your patient, how much cuff pressure should you use?

A. Up to 200 mm HG

B. Until you no longer hear a pulse

C. Up to 100- 200 mm HG, depending on the size of the patient

D. 30 mm Hg above the point at which the pulse disappears

XXXXXDXXXXX

6. When the nurse requests that you get a rectal temperature on a patient she suspects has a fever, how do you obtain this?

A. Use an electric thermometer under the arm

B. Use a paper thermometer on the forehead

C. Use a designated thermometer with a red probe, inserted into the rectum

D. Use the same thermometer you use for all patients, inserted under the tongue

XXXXXCXXXXX

7. What should you do when you are attempting to obtain a blood pressure on an obese patient and the blood pressure cuff will not fit all the way around the patients arm?

A. Switch to a larger cuff

B. Attempt the blood pressure on the leg

C. Just write down what the blood pressure was the last time it was taken

D. Ask the patient what his blood pressure normally runs, and record that as the blood pressure

XXXXXAXXXXX

8. When your patient's blood pressure is 115/75, what does the upper number represent?

A. The diastolic pressure

B. The heart rate

C. The patient's age

D. The systolic pressure

XXXXXDXXXXX

9. What should you do when you enter your patient's room to obtain a blood pressure and realize the patient has an IV infusing to the left arm?

A. Take the blood pressure from the left arm

B. Wait until the IV is removed to get the blood pressure

C. Take the blood pressure from the right arm

D. Use the smallest possible cuff

XXXXXCXXXXX

10. How long and what should you watch for when counting the respiratory rate on a patient?

A. Do not allow the patient to talk while you are counting

B. Watch the rise and fall of the chest a minimum of thirty seconds

C. Watch the clock and listen for respirations

D. Ask the patient to hold her breath

XXXXXBXXXXX

Made in United States
Orlando, FL
22 February 2022

15058201R00135